Being a Medical Records/Health Information Clerk

PRENTICE HALL HEALTH MEDICAL CLERICAL SERIES
Kay Cox-Stevens, RN, MA, Series Editor

Being a Medical Clerical Worker: An Introductory Core Text, *Jacquelyn Marshall, BA, MT, MA*

Being a Medical Records/Health Information Clerk, *Kathryn McMiller, RHIA*

Being a Medical Insurance Coder, *Laurie Dodson, RHIA, MPH*

Kay Cox-Stevens, RN, MA, is a Health Careers Specialist, Medical Assistant Program Coordinator at Saddleback College; and author of Prentice Hall's *Being a Health Unit Coordinator*.

Being a Medical Records/Health Information Clerk

Third Edition

Kathryn McMiller, RHIA

Kay Cox-Stevens, RN, MA
Series Editor

PEARSON

Prentice Hall

Upper Saddle River, New Jersey 07458

Library of Congress Cataloging-in-Publication Data

McMiller, Kathryn.
  Being a medical records/health information clerk / Kathryn McMiller.—
3rd ed.
      p. ; cm. — (Prentice Hall Health medical clerical series)
Rev. ed. of: Being a medical records clerk. 2nd ed. c2000.
Includes bibliographical references (p.   ) and index.
  ISBN 0-13-112671-7
  1. Medical records personnel. 2. Medical records—Management.
  [DNLM: 1. Medical Records. 2. Confidentiality. 3. Information
Management. 4. Medical Record Administrators. WX 173 M478b 2003] I.
McMiller, Kathryn. Being a medical records clerk. II. Title. III.
Series.
  RA976.5 .M38 2004
  651.5'04261—dc21

                                    2003004420

Notice

Care has been taken to confirm the accuracy of the information presented in this book. The author, editor, and the publisher, however, cannot accept any responsibility for errors or omissions or for the consequences for application of the information in this book and make no warranty, express or implied, with respect to its contents.

The author and publisher disclaim all responsibility for any liability, loss, injury, or damage incurred as a consequence, directly or indirectly, of the use and application of any of the contents of this volume.

Publisher: Julie Levin Alexander
Assistant to Publisher: Regina Bruno
Executive Editor: Barbara Krawiec
Editorial Assistant: Sheba Jalaluddin
Director of Production and Manufacturing: Bruce Johnson
Managing Production Editor: Patrick Walsh
Production Liaison: Mary C. Treacy
Production Editor: Jessica Balch, Pine Tree Composition
Manufacturing Manager: Ilene Sanford

Manufacturing Buyer: Pat Brown
Design Director: Cheryl Asherman
Cover Designer: Chris Weigand
Senior Marketing Manager: Nicole Benson
Marketing Assistant: Janet Ryerson
Channel Information Manager: Rachele Strober
Composition: Pine Tree Composition, Inc.
Printer/Binder: Banta Book Group
Cover Printer: Phoenix Color Corp.

Pearson Education Ltd., *London*
Pearson Education Australia Pty. Limited, *Sydney*
Pearson Education Singapore, Pte. Ltd.
Pearson Education North Asia Ltd., *Hong Kong*
Pearson Education Canada, Ltd., *Toronto*
Pearson Educación de Mexico, S.A. de C.V.
Pearson Education—Japan, *Tokyo*
Pearson Education Malaysia, Pte. Ltd.
Pearson Education, *Upper Saddle River, New Jersey*

1 0 9 8 7 6 5
ISBN 0-13-112671-7

To My Parents
Keith and Jane
for their constant love
and encouragement

Contents

Foreword

Choosing a medical clerical career is a smart decision. The U.S. Bureau of Labor and Statistics reports medical clerical occupations to be one of the fastest growing through 2010. Some of the reasons for the continuing demand for medical clerical workers include the aging of America and the rapid increase in the number of medical tests and treatments available. The resultant paperwork requires workers trained to maintain medical records and select and apply codes for insurance billing and statistics gathering. Legal considerations and the scrutiny of managed care, Medicare, third-party payers, regulators, the courts, and consumers have made the proper management of patient's charts increasingly important.

Industry, on the other hand, reports that there are not nearly enough trained medical clerical workers to meet the demand and many jobs go unfilled. Adequate training opportunities and training tools are in short supply, particularly in some career areas.

The Prentice Hall Health Medical Clerical Series was created in recognition of these needs. Designed as easy-to-understand yet comprehensive texts, this series guides students through the duties and responsibilities of medical clerical workers in their chosen fields. *Being a Medical Clerical Worker: An Introductory Core Text* contains information considered common to all medical clerical areas. This book, *Being a Medical Records/Health Information Clerk* is written for students interested in working in health information management.

It is hoped that this series will make a significant contribution toward filling the gap of supply and demand for medical clerical workers and that you, the student, will utilize these books to the fullest degree as you embark on your new career.

Kay Cox-Stevens
Series Editor

Preface

As the requirements for more and diverse types of documentation in medical records increase, the role of the Medical Records/Health Information Clerk in keeping the Health Information Management Department functioning becomes more and more critical. It is the intent of this text to provide basic information that will make the entry-level Medical Records/Health Information Clerk immediately effective.

Chapters 1 and 2 provide an overview of the Medical Records/Health Information Clerk function and the Health Information Management Department. Chapters 3, 4, 5, and 6 teach the student filing and retrieval, record processing, assembly, and analysis. Chapter 7 discusses working with physicians in the Physician Incomplete Area. Chapter 8 deals with confidentiality and release of information, and Chapter 9 discusses other functions to which a Medical Records/Health Information Clerk may be assigned. Each chapter discusses computerization of documentation and the functions of a Health Information Management Department, where applicable.

The text of *Being a Medical Records/Health Information Clerk* is designed to be used as a reference. Each chapter begins with a vocabulary of pertinent terms used in the chapter and specific objectives of the subject matter. Frequent headings and subheadings are identified throughout each chapter. The summary reviews the main points of the chapter. Learning activities at the end of each chapter give the student an opportunity to put into use the ideas discussed.

Examples and opinions expressed as to the most effective means of performing a function are the author's opinion based on training, experience, and networking with colleagues. Methods for performing health information management functions vary based on individual Health Information Management Department demands, and no attempt has been made to illustrate all methods.

ACKNOWLEDGMENTS

The author wishes to express her sincere thanks to those individuals who assisted in preparing this text.

- Kay Cox-Stevens, Medical Clerical Series Editor, who gave me encouragement and a push when I procrastinated.
- Lois Miller, who helped develop the original outline, and Verda Weston, who provided criticism and encouragement.
- Rose Anderson, Patricia Hudson, Frances Gonzales, and Roberta Whitson for providing information about medical record practice in Colorado, Florida, Texas, and Oklahoma.
- Gina Gomez and Linda Fenstermaker, who deciphered my handwriting and dictation to type the first draft of the manuscript.
- Cheryl Servais, who offered empathy, ideas, and constructive criticism.
- The Health Information Services Department staff of Placentia Linda Hospital, Placentia, California, for being Medical Records/Health Information Clerk role models.
- Rosalie Janish, Cypress, California, who provided a review.

- Lisa Robinson, Beth Zallar, Tanya Aigner, Lynn Bree, Marie Serrao, and Verda Weston, who gave me assistance in updating various sections.
- Paul Martinez at Versatile Information Products for the digital dictation system illustration.
- LaDonna Thomason at St. John Record Programs, Inc., for the file folder illustration.

Kathryn McMiller

ABOUT THE AUTHOR

Kathryn McMiller, RHIA, is an independent Health Information Management consultant based in Southern California. She has over 24 years experience in HIM, the last eight years as a consultant specializing in interim HIM department assessments and interim management and computer system installation project management. Kathryn has worked in hospitals ranging in size from 110 to 1,000 beds in various parts of the country.

ABOUT THE SERIES EDITOR

Kay Cox-Stevens, RN, MA is Program Coordinator of the Medical Assistant Program at Saddleback College in Mission Viejo, California, and owner of Achiever's Development Enterprises, a consulting and publishing business. She is a former Professional Development Consultant for Special Projects and Curriculum Development for the California Department of Education. She was a Master Trainer for Health Careers Teacher Training through California Polytechnic University of Pomona and served as chairperson of the California Health Careers Statewide Advisory Committee. She was a critical care nurse and inservice educator. Professor Cox-Stevens conceived this series and worked with the authors to develop each book.

Being a Medical Records/Health Information Clerk

Assembly	Arranging the documents of the medical record in a specified order after discharge of the patient.
Authorization	A signed consent of the patient or his or her representative to release confidential information.
Compromise care	To make the patient's care less effective.
Contract service	A company hired to perform a function when the health information management department is unable to manage the amount of work, such as transcription of dictation.
Discharge summary	A report, dictated by a physician at the end of hospitalization, that details the diagnoses and treatment given.
Health information management department	The department, in a healthcare facility, responsible for maintaining security and confidentiality of patient records and for promoting responsible use of the records in patient care.
Indexing	Assigning a document to the correct patient, document type, and episode of care in an optical imaging system.
Loose documents	Documents received by the health information management department, after the patient has been discharged, that must be placed in the record.
Medical record	A multiform document detailing the patient's diagnoses, diagnostic testing, and treatment given during an encounter with the hospital. Portions of the record may be computerized.
Medical transcription	Interpretation and typing of reports dictated by physicians and other healthcare personnel.
Misfile	To file a record or document in the wrong location.
Operative report	A report dictated by the surgeon detailing the surgical procedure and findings.
Optical imaging system	A computer system in which documents are converted to computer images that can be viewed simultaneously by multiple users.
Quality control	Review of documents that have been scanned into an optical imaging system to insure that they are legible and have been indexed correctly.
Scanning	The process of converting a paper document into a computer image.

When you have completed this chapter, you will be able to:

- Describe three characteristics desirable in a medical records/HIM clerk and why.
- Describe four functions a medical records/HIM clerk may perform in the health information management department.
- Relate the career opportunities available through the health information management department.

*I*NTRODUCTION

Being a medical records/health information (HIM) clerk can be a rewarding position for the person who is detail-oriented, a quick worker, and interested in quality. Career opportunities are numerous and career goals can be reached with prerequisite years of education and work experience.

*J*OB PREREQUISITES

Medical records/HIM clerks can be employed in acute care hospitals, long-term care hospitals specializing in rehabilitation and convalescence, nursing homes, physician offices, ambulatory care settings, and temporary service agencies.

A medical records/HIM clerk is usually an entry-level position in a **health information management (HIM) department.** As with any position, the department director would like to hire a clerk with experience; however, because experienced clerks are not easy to find, the prerequisites for an entry-level medical records/HIM clerk are minimal (Figure 1.1).

Education

A high school diploma or equivalent is necessary to ensure that you have the basic knowledge needed to learn this new job. Typing is essential both for computer entry as well as typed data. Alphabetical filing is the most basic of filing systems. If you can perform it successfully, it should be easy for you to learn the numerical filing systems always found in an HIM department.

Communication Skills

Health information management departments communicate daily with patients, other department personnel, physician office workers, and, especially, physicians. It is necessary that you have good communication skills to function effectively. This means that you can listen and take notes accurately; ask appropriate questions, if the information is not clear; and speak slowly and clearly.

Initiative

The person who is willing to learn new things and takes the initiative to do so always has an advantage over one who waits to be told what to do. There is always work to be done in an HIM department.

```
– High school graduate or equivalent
– Type 40–45 wpm
– Ability to alphabetize data
– Good communication skills
– Self-confidence, initiative, and willingness to learn
```

FIGURE 1.1 Prerequisites for becoming a medical records/HIM clerk.

𝓜EDICAL RECORDS/HIM CLERK FUNCTIONS

File Clerk

The opportunities for an entry-level medical records/HIM clerk vary from department to department. You may start out as a file clerk assigned to the permanent file area. Your responsibilities will include pulling records that have been requested, filing **loose documents** into the correct **medical records,** and refiling records that have been returned to the department (Figure 1.2). Accuracy is extremely important. If you **misfile** a record, you may be able to find it again, but only after a time-consuming search. If you misfile a document, it may be lost forever unless someone accidentally discovers it in the wrong record.

In the meantime, that misfiled record or document may delay or prevent billing so that the hospital does not get paid. More important, lost information can **compromise** the quality of the patient's **care.** If the attending physician cannot refer to the record to obtain information about previous hospitalizations, operations, and diagnostic tests, the patient may have to undergo those tests again or be exposed to an anesthetic or drug to which he or she is allergic. The proper filing of the medical record is extremely important to the smooth operation of the medical record department and the entire hospital.

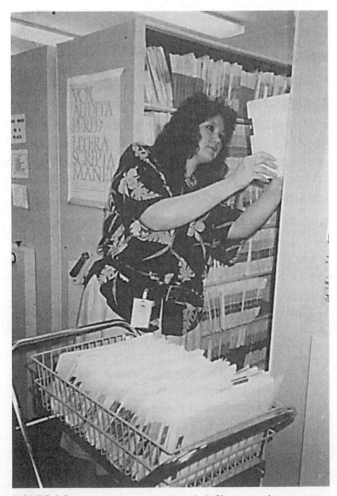

FIGURE 1.2 A medical records/HIM clerk filing records.

Other Entry-Level Duties

In other departments, the entry-level medical records/HIM clerk may have other duties in addition to filing. The medical records/HIM clerk may create file folders for new patients or pick up the records of discharged patients from nursing units. With further training and time on the job, the medical records/HIM clerk may **assemble** records into final format and analyze them for missing physician signatures and documentation such as **operative reports** and **discharge summaries.** A similar function involves **scanning** documents into an **optical imaging system** and performing **indexing** and **quality control.**

Birth Certificates

Some medical records/HIM clerks process birth certificates by interviewing the mothers, typing the certificates, obtaining signatures, and maintaining a birth log.

Release of Information

The medical records/HIM clerk may be trained to release information upon written authorization from the patient or other third party in accordance with state and federal regulations. Some medical records/HIM clerks are trained to answer telephone requests for information.

Physician Incomplete Area

Working with the physicians in the physician incomplete area is another function that may be performed by a medical records/HIM clerk. This area is where physicians come to complete the omissions of signatures and documentation identified during record analysis.

CAREER OPPORTUNITIES

Although being a medical records/HIM clerk is an interesting job, you may be wondering what career opportunities are available. The career opportunities for a medical records/HIM clerk are many and diverse.

Senior Medical Records/Health Information Clerk

In the health information management department (Figure 1.3) you can advance to senior medical records/HIM clerk, or Technician II. Senior medical records/HIM clerks perform the advanced clerical functions such as analysis and working in the physician incomplete area, which we discussed previously. Medical records/HIM clerks and senior clerks are called Technicians I and II in some departments. Titles vary across the country.

Registered Health Information Technician

From senior clerk you could attend a two-year course, usually offered at a community college, to prepare to become a registered health information technician (RHIT). The program requires performing tasks in an actual hospital health information management department. Upon successful completion of an RHIT program, you may take a national examination. Passing the examination allows you to use the credential of RHIT. As an RHIT you can be a coder, a cancer registrar, a supervisor, or an assistant or associate HIM department director in a large hospital. With addi-

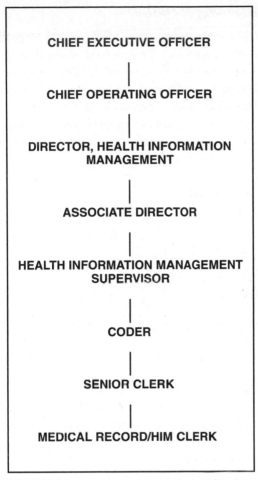

FIGURE 1.3 Career ladder through the health information management department.

tional work experience or education, some RHITs also become health information management department directors.

Registered Health Information Administrator

If you decide that management of an HIM department is your goal, you may undertake a four-year college course or a graduate program to become a registered health information administrator (RHIA). RHIAs may be supervisors, assistant HIM department directors, or directors. With additional education, such as a master's degree in business administration or public health, and work experience, a department director may be promoted to an administrative level within the facility.

RHIAs may become performance improvement or case managers. Or, they can work for accounting firms that monitor the efficiency of healthcare facility departments.

Consultant

RHITs and RHIAs with experience may go into HIM consulting, which offers a variety of job experiences. Firms specializing in HIM consulting provide a range of services including coding, HIM department review and assessment, implementation of computer systems, and interim HIM department management. Some of these firms also provide temporary employees when departments have staff vacancies or backlogs in work. Many HIM consulting firms are owned by HIM professionals.

Certified Coding Specialist

The American Health Information Management Association (AHIMA) offers a national examination for anyone with coding experience or education to become a Certified Coding Specialist (CCS). Many community colleges offer courses leading to a coding certificate and the ability to write the CCS exam. Most hospitals prefer that a coder have the CCS credential.

Educator

Both RHITs and RHIAs can become teachers of college-level HIM courses or conduct seminars for continuing education.

PROFESSIONAL AFFILIATION

If you decide that a career in health information management is your goal, you can become a student member of AHIMA while pursuing your RHIT or RHIA education. Student members are often given the opportunity to attend state and national association meetings for a nominal charge. Your department director will be able to give you the information necessary to contact AHIMA, or you can visit the Web site at *www.AHIMA.org*.

With AHIMA membership, you automatically become a member of your state HIM association. Many state associations send out monthly publications to keep members informed about the latest changes in law, equipment, and other items that affect the medical records field. These associations also offer workshops throughout the year to help members obtain continuing education (CE) hours that are required to maintain an RHIT or RHIA credential.

MEDICAL TRANSCRIPTION

It is possible for a medical records clerk to become a **medical transcriptionist.** Programs in a variety of educational settings offer the necessary courses including use of word processors or computer software and extensive medical terminology. Transcriptionists can work in the HIM department or in separate transcription units in radiology, cardiology, or pathology. Many transcriptionists work exclusively for physicians and specialize in one type of transcription, such as orthopedics. A transcriptionist may work for or own a contract service. **Contract services** transcribe for departments with vacancies or a sudden increase in the amount of dictation received. Many hospitals have no employed transcriptionists and use a contract service for all transcription.

SUMMARY

The opportunities for the medical records/health information (HIM) clerk in hospitals and other healthcare settings are diverse. The extent of your career as a medical records/HIM clerk and beyond will be determined by your own initiative, perseverance, and drive.

*L*EARNING ACTIVITIES

1. Name and discuss three characteristics desirable in a medical records/ HIM clerk.

2. What is AHIMA and what significance does it have to a career in HIM?

3. Name five functions in a medical records department to which a medical records/HIM clerk may be assigned.

4. Describe the difference between the RHIT and RHIA credentials and discuss the possible career opportunities for each.

5. Surf the AHIMA Web site and report on at least five resources AHIMA provides to its members.

The Health Information Management Department

VOCABULARY

Abstracting   Collection of data from the medical record for statistical and planning purposes.

Analysis   Reviewing the medical record to determine that all required documentation is present including signatures and reports.

Cancer registry   A database of patients diagnosed with cancer.

Coding   Assignment of numbers to diagnoses and/or procedures using the current edition of a coding or classification system such as the International Classification of Diseases (ICD) or Current Procedural Terminology (CPT).

Deficiency slip   A document that identifies deficiencies in documentation.

Healthcare provider   An individual or facility, such as a hospital, that provides healthcare to a patient.

JCAHO   Joint Commission on the Accreditation of Healthcare Organizations.

Litigation   Lawsuit.

Medical record number   A unique number assigned to a medical record in order to identify it.

Medical transcription   Interpretation and typing of reports dictated by physicians and other healthcare personnel.

Medicare   Federal insurance for patients over 65 or for the disabled.

Performance improvement   Evaluating the overall performance of a healthcare facility, from the environment to patient care, with the purpose of continuous improvement.

Periodical   A magazine or journal published at specified periods, for example, weekly or monthly.

Physician incomplete area   Area of the health information management department where physicians come to work on incomplete records.

Physician progress note   Handwritten or typed entries made by the physician regarding the patient's progress during hospitalization or other treatment.

Risk management   Addressing the risk to which patients, visitors, hospital staff, medical staff, vendors, and others are exposed.

Third party   A person or entity, such as an insurance company, other than the healthcare facility or patient.

OBJECTIVES

When you have completed this chapter you will be able to:

- Describe the different purposes for maintaining a medical record.
- Name the basic job functions found in the health information management department and discuss their relationship to the medical record.
- Name three functions that may be performed in the health information management department.

$\mathcal{U}$ SES OF A MEDICAL RECORD

In the early years of medical documentation, the record of a patient's stay in the hospital usually consisted of one line in a ledger which gave the patient's name, address, chief complaint, the doctor's name, the amount paid, and possibly a few lines about the type of treatment given. In 1928, the American Medical Record Association (AMRA) was founded to promote standards for the accuracy and quality of patient care documentation. The name was later changed to American Health Information Management Association (AHIMA) in an effort to recognize the changing roles of HIM professionals in managing health information that no longer consisted of a paper record only. The medical record has evolved from a ledger line entry to a complex multiform document containing computer-generated data. Some portions or all of the record may be created and stored on other types of media such as videotape, microfilm, and computers.

Patient Care

The medical record has multiple uses. Primarily, it is a document of the evaluation and treatment received by the patient during a healthcare encounter, whether it be as an inpatient, as an outpatient, or in an emergency room. The record documents communication between the physician who is responsible for the patient's treatment and the hospital professional personnel who assist in caring for the patient. These personnel include nurses, pharmacists, therapists, dieticians, and other professionals. The communication takes the form of physician orders and the response to those orders as documented in **physician progress notes** and diagnostic test results. The information in a medical record should be documented as accurately and as thoroughly as possible so that the next **healthcare provider** treating the patient can continue treatment without having to reschedule diagnostic tests or other treatment.

Legal Document

In all states, the medical record is considered a legal document. It can be used as evidence in a court of law (**litigation**). The basic legal tenet of record keeping is that "if it isn't documented, it didn't happen." This is important, especially in malpractice cases. The physician being sued may state that he or she conducted a certain course of treatment or that the patient refused the treatment offered. But, if the physician has not documented this information in the record, it is likely that the jury will not believe that the treatment or refusal occurred. Thorough and accurate documentation protects the patient, the hospital, and the physician.

Statistics

A third purpose for the medical record is its use in collection of data for research. The records of patients being treated for a disease may be studied to determine trends in response or lack of response to different treatment modalities. Forms can be developed for use in the record so that the information is collected in the same manner for each patient. This standardization makes correlation of statistical data much easier and more accurate. These statistics are used to change or support a particular type of treatment. Codes assigned to diseases and procedures can also be used for statistical compilation.

Other Uses

Other uses of the medical record include substantiating billing charges, teaching, and performance improvement. **Coding** and **performance improvement,** which use documentation found in the record, will be discussed later in this chapter.

HEALTH INFORMATION MANAGEMENT DEPARTMENT FUNCTIONS

Now that we have examined the different uses for the medical record, let's look at the functions that are performed in the health information management department so that the record is available for those purposes. The first function is storage and retrieval.

Storage and Retrieval

In order for a medical record to be available for the many uses described above, it must be filed in a way so that the information is secure and remains confidential but can be retrieved easily. The medical record itself consists of documents accumulated during the patient's course of treatment. These documents are normally stored in a manila file folder which is assigned a **medical record number.** Usually, each patient is given one medical record number at a particular healthcare facility. The various ways of assigning numbers will be discussed later. The manila folders themselves are normally filed on open shelves.

Most HIM departments have a policy that only department personnel may enter the file area and pull records. Such a policy exists so that confidentiality is maintained and so that records are not taken by unauthorized personnel. It also allows the department to maintain control over the records. As we discussed in Chapter 1, if a record is misfiled or misplaced, the patient's care may be compromised.

Some departments have computer systems that enable them to track the location of individual records. Most allow for bar coding of each individual record. Then the record may be checked out with the use of a barcode reader like those you find in grocery stores to enter the item in the cash register.

Because most health information management departments have a space shortage, it eventually becomes necessary to examine alternative means of storing older records. Some departments microfilm records and use a microfilm reader/printer to view the records when a patient is readmitted or to reconstruct the filmed record on paper. Because this is a very expensive procedure, many facilities have decided to store the records off site, at a separate location, instead of microfilming. Some states, such as California, have requirements as to the type of structure required to store records off site. The facility must be secure, must be fireproof, and must provide 24-hour-a-day retrieval of the records. Records may also be stored in an optical imaging system, where the paper documents are scanned and converted into digital data. Scanned images are stored on platters in a "juke box" and are viewed on a computer monitor.

Release of Information

The release of information function involves receiving a request for information about a particular patient and responding to that request. The request may be in writing or it may be verbal. It may come from the patient, a physician office, a **third-party** payer, or another healthcare provider. The employee performing the release of information function has a primary responsibility to protect the confidentiality of the patient information. Most states have regulations regarding what information may be released without a patient's consent. The federal government has regulations regarding the release of information pertaining to treatment of drug and alcohol abuse. The medical records/HIM clerk must receive the request, determine if the requester is authorized to receive the information, pull the record, determine if the information requested is available from the medical record, copy that information, and forward it to the requesting party. Many HIM departments utilize the services of contract copy services. These services bring their own employees into the department to copy the medical record and mail it to the requester.

Coding

One of the most important functions of the HIM department is diagnostic and procedural coding. This function is usually performed by accredited record technicians (RHITs) or clinical coding specialists (CCSs) who have been trained in using the current editions of the International Classification of Diseases (ICD) (Figure 2.1) and Current Procedural Terminology (CPT). ICD is a system developed to classify numerically all of the different diseases that a patient might be treated for and all of the different diagnostic and surgical procedures used in the treatment of a particular disease process. It was originally developed to provide statistical data regarding the causes of death throughout the world, and it is still used for this purpose to a certain extent. It is also used to determine incidence of disease. CPT is a system designed by the American Medical Association to classify all of the procedures performed on a patient in a physician office. In the United States, coding is done primarily for reimbursement.

The Centers for Medicare and Medicaid Services (CMS) uses ICD and CPT to determine the payment that a hospital receives for treating **Medicare** inpatients and outpatients. If a coder fails to select the correct codes, there may be a resulting decrease in the amount of reimbursement that the hospital is entitled to. In order to code a record accurately, a coder must understand all of the documentation in the medical record, including laboratory and diagnostic test results, and be able to work with the physician to insure that all diagnoses and procedures are documented as accurately as possible.

Corporate Compliance

Inaccurate coding can lead to decreased reimbursement for a hospital, but it can also lead to increased reimbursement not supported by the medical record documentation. The federal government considers this to be fraud and estimates it loses millions

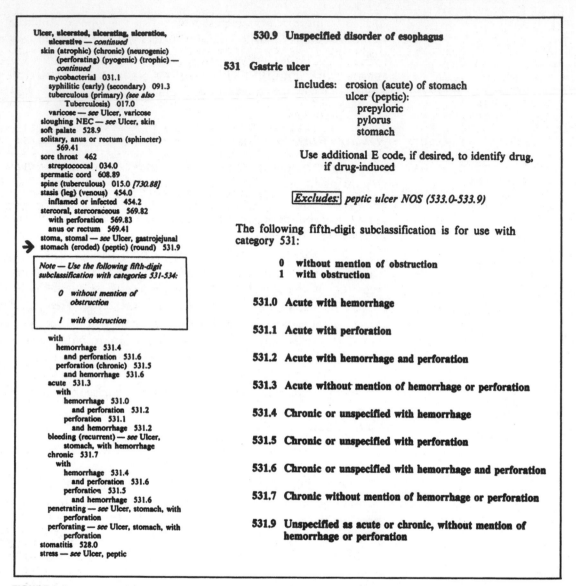

FIGURE 2.1 Example of ICD-9-CM Alphabetical Index and Tabular List. To code a stomach ulcer, the coder would search the index (left) for the entry (see arrow). Once the correct description is found, the coder goes to the Tabular List (right) to determine the correct code.

of dollars every year because of fraudulent coding. Consequently, each hospital is required to have a corporate compliance program in place.

A corporate compliance plan program requires that all employees are trained in recognizing irregular or fraudulent practices and given opportunities for reporting them without fear of reprisal. Coders must sign that they have been trained and will not engage in fraudulent coding. Yearly, the hospital must also show evidence of continuing education of current coding practices for each coder.

Abstracting

Another function usually done in conjunction with coding, is **abstracting**. This is a procedure for collecting (abstracting) information from the medical record and entering it into a computer program. The abstract (Figure 2.2) contains spaces (fields) that are specified for individual pieces of information. For example, one field may contain the patient's last name, another field may contain the first name, and another

```
                              HOSPITAL      ABSTRACT MAINTENANCE
ABS STS: C COMPLETE     COMP DT:  2/10/  LST MNT:  2/11/  PRT BILL SH:  (Y/N)
------------------------------ DEMOGRAPHIC DATA ------------------------------
MED.REC.#   ACCT. # PATIENT LAST NAME        FIRST NAME       PERSONAL I.D.
   178360  2776623
LOCAL ADDRESS              CITY           ST ZIP CODE +4     DNR ORDER
     WOODWIND LN.          ANAHEIM        CA                 ***
D.O.B.     AGE      SEX      DIAG/PROC EDITS RACE        ET  MARITAL STATUS
05261924  74 YEARS  F FEMALE AGE: Y SEX: Y  1 WHITE      3   M MARRIED
------------------------------ VISIT SUMMARY ------------------------------
PATIENT TYPE     DAY CARE  PRIMARY FINANCIAL CLASS  SECONDARY FINANCIAL CLASS
1 INPATIENT                80 PPA
PATIENT SOURCE   ADMISSION TYPE    HSP SRV 42 DEFINITIVE OBSE  SEEN IN ED   Y
A PHYSICIAN       3 NECESSARY           ARRIVAL                LIC LVL CAR  3
          DATE    TIME  ACCOMMODATION ISO   L.O.S.
INITIAL REG:  0205           24 DEFICU          2       RE-ADMIT
ADMISSION:    0205  1556 24 DEFICU VFY STAY:   (Y)      FOLLOWUP
DISCHARGE:    0207  0945      CORONER AUTP   DTH-LOS ANES     POST-OP   IN O.R.
A HOME/SELF          N       N (Y/N) N (Y/N) N (Y/N) N (Y/N)  N (Y/N)   N (Y/N)
TOTAL CHARGES:   1197049     DEPT: M  MED SRV: 10   MEDICINE (GENERAL)   VFY


  KEY IN/CHANGE THE INFORMATION SHOWN ABOVE; THEN PRESS ENTER FOR AN EDIT.
F4=EOT  F6=PRV SCRN  F7=EOJ  F8=RESTRT  F9=HELP  F2=ZIP           F15=TABLE INQ
```

```
                         HOSPITAL      ABSTRACT MAINTENANCE
MED.REC.#:    178360  ACCT. #: 2776623  PATIENT NAME:

              MF PA  CODE      DESCRIPTION
ADMITTING DX:        578.9     GASTROINTEST HEMORR
-----------------------------------------------------------------------------
PRINCIPAL DX:     Y  578.9     GASTROINTEST HEMORR
-----------------------------------------------------------------------------
ADDITIONAL DIAGNOSES:
   MF PA CODE     DESCRIPTION        MF PA CODE     DESCRIPTION
  2:    Y V45.1   RENAL DIALYSIS STAT  3:  Y 276.5   HYPOVOLEMIA
  4:    Y 403.91  HYPERT REN DIS NOS   5:  Y 412     OLD MYOCARDIAL INFA
  6:    Y 272.0   PURE HYPERCHOLESTER  7:  Y 535.50  GASTRITIS/DUODENITI
  8:    Y 530.19  ESOPHAGITIS, NEC     9:  Y 530.81  ESOPHAGEAL REFLUX
 10:    Y 414.01  CORONARY ATHERO, NA 11:  Y V12.72  PERSONAL HX COLONIC
 12:    Y 787.01  NAUSEA WITH VOMITIN 13:  Y 787.91  DIARRHEA
 14:                                  15:


TOTAL FINAL DIAGNOSES: 13    INTERFACE: 3        M.D.C.:   6  D.R.G.:  174
STILLBORN:        HOSPITAL COMPLICATION: N (Y/N)  HOSPITAL INFECTION: N (Y/N)

  KEY IN/CHANGE THE INFORMATION SHOWN ABOVE; THEN PRESS ENTER FOR AN EDIT.
F3=DRG MSG F4=EOT F5=AHFS INQ F6=PRV SCRN F7=EOJ F8=RESTART F9=HELP F11=DX INQ
F13=DSPMSG    F14=SNDMSG    F15=TBL INQ      F23=INT-FCE  F24=E.D. DIAGNOSIS
```

FIGURE 2.2 An example of three screens of a computerized abstract used to collect data from the medical record.

field may contain the patient's medical record number. Types of information that are collected include the identification numbers for the different physicians who have treated the patient, the number of days that a patient may have been cared for on a special unit such as the intensive care unit, the disposition of the patient on discharge, and the patient's age and sex.

The information collected from the abstracts is stored in a computer database from which statistical reports are generated. Hospitals use these reports to determine

```
                          HOSPITAL        ABSTRACT MAINTENANCE
MED.REC.#:     178360  ACCT. #: 2776623  PATIENT NAME:
------------------------------- PROCEDURE DATA -------------------------------
     MF  PROCEDURE CODE/DESC        DATE     SURGEON NUMBER/NAME    EPISODE #
PRIN-    UHDDS    ANESTHESIA TYPE/DESC    TISSUE TYPE/DESC      ABN RSLT
CIPAL:   45.16    EGD WITH CLOSED BIO 020699  01022
         1        1 NONE

   2:


   3:


   4:


   5:


   TOTAL PROCEDURES: 01                ADDITIONAL PROCEDURES: NO
 KEY IN/CHANGE THE INFORMATION SHOWN ABOVE; THEN PRESS ENTER FOR AN EDIT.
F4=EOT          F6=PRV SCREEN        F7=EOJ               F8=RESTART
F9=HELP         F10=DOCTOR INQUIRY   F11=PROC. INQUIRY    F13=DSPMSG
F14=SNDMSG      F15=TABLE INQ.       F22=CORRECT EPISODE #  F23=INTERFACE
```

FIGURE 2.2 Continued.

the utilization of the hospital by different physicians, to determine staffing needs, and to supply data required by government agencies. Government agencies use the information to get an overall picture of healthcare utilization by county and by state. This helps with funding for medical care and planning for the future.

$\mathcal{A}$ SSEMBLY AND ANALYSIS

Assembly

Assembly of the medical record is a function that a medical records/HIM clerk performs when the patient is discharged from the healthcare facility. The medical record is removed from the binder where it has been kept on the nursing station and is taken to the health information management department.

Chart Order List

Every hospital has a specified order (chart order list) in which the documents that make up the medical record are arranged. This order may vary from facility to facility depending on the needs of the hospital medical staff and employees.

In many cases the chart order is a universal chart order, meaning that the same chart order is used for the medical record on the nursing unit and in the medical record file folder after the patient is discharged.

To maintain the universal chart order, multiple dividers are used in the nursing unit record. Some hospitals use paper dividers with reinforced tabs that are removed from the binder with the documents after patient discharge and then placed in the file folder in HIM. Others use the paper dividers, but to save money, recycle them back to the nursing units at the time of assembly. Plastic dividers that remain in the nursing unit binders are also used.

The medical records/HIM clerk doing assembly uses the chart order list as a reference in spot checking that documents are in the correct order. Documents are usually left in the order in which they are received from the nursing unit. This means that the documents are in reverse chronological order, with the newest document on the top of each section for easy reference. Occasionally, a few documents will be moved to a new location in the file folder. For example, the facesheet may be moved to the top of the record so that the particular episode of care can be easily identified in the file folder.

MR # _____

CHART DEFICIENCY SLIP

	DICTATE/COMPLETE	SIGN
Face Sheet	_____	_____
Discharge Summary	_____	_____
Condition on Disch.	_____	_____
Final Diagnosis	_____	_____
History & Physical	_____	_____
Consultation	_____	_____
Progress Notes	_____	_____
Pre-op Prog. Note	_____	_____
Post-op Prog. Note	_____	_____
Operative Report	_____	_____
Physician Orders	_____	_____

Other:_____

_____

_____

PATIENT NAME _____ DISCH. DATE _____

PHYSICIAN _____

FIGURE 2.3 An example of a manual lack/deficiency slip.

Some hospitals reassemble the entire record into the chart order, including placing each section of documents in chronological order. This practice depends on the volume of patients and the number of staff available in HIM.

Analysis

Analysis of the record is sometimes done in conjunction with assembly or it can be done as a separate function. The analysis clerk reviews each document in the record to ensure that it belongs to the correct patient. Analysis also involves reviewing each page of the record to ensure that all entries are signed by physicians and other caregivers and to ensure that all reports that should be dictated, such as operative reports, history and physical examinations, consultation reports, and discharge summaries, have been dictated. When an omission is found, it is noted. A **deficiency slip** (Figure 2.3) is generated for each individual physician who must complete some portion of the record. There are various methods for doing this and we will discuss them later in the text. Analysis of the record must be done in a timely manner to meet various regulations and laws. The **Joint Commission on the Accreditation of Healthcare Organizations (JCAHO)** requires that all records be complete within 30 days of patient discharge. Some state governments also have regulations regarding the completion of records. For example, in California, the record must be completed within fourteen days of discharge. Consequently, the record must be analyzed quickly so that physicians and others are given a sufficient amount of time to meet the completion regulations.

$\mathcal{T}$RANSCRIPTION

Transcription involves taking the spoken word and turning it into a printed document. The physician may dictate a report from his or her office, from somewhere in the hospital, or possibly from a cellular phone. The report is recorded on the hospital's or a contracted vendor's digital dictation system and then transcribed using word processing software specifically designed for **medical transcription.**

Dictation and transcription systems are usually interfaced. As soon as the transcriptionist begins transcribing, the demographic data entered by the physician using the telephone keypad is automatically entered into the report. This saves the transcriptionist time and reduces errors.

When the dictation is recorded and transcribed on a vendor's systems, the reports are electronically imported into the hospital's computer system and then printed.

Digital dictation systems have management software that tracks the dictation by date and time of dictation, report type, and person doing the dictating. These systems can be set up to route reports to each transcriptionist automatically. Different reports are given different priorities for typing. For example, history and physical (H&P) and consultation reports are given priority over discharge summaries and operative reports, because the information contained in the H&P and consultation is needed immediately to treat the patient. This also holds true for procedure reports and any other diagnostic test reports. Once the report priority has been established, the next rule in a transcription area is that of "first in, first out," meaning that the oldest dictation is always done first.

Medical transcription requires an extensive knowledge of both medical terminology and clinical disease processes. It is not only important to know how to spell the words, but the transcriptionist must also be able to interpret from the context of the report which words the physician is referring to, because physicians rarely spell the words. There are many medical words that sound exactly alike but are spelled differently and have different meanings (e.g., *ilium* and *ileum*). The transcriptionist must be able to determine from the content of the dictation whether the doctor is talking about the hip (*ilium*) or small intestine (*ileum*); otherwise, he or she may use the wrong word and make the report inaccurate.

COMPLETION OF MEDICAL RECORDS

Once the medical record has been analyzed it is placed into the **physician incomplete area.** The record remains here until all caregivers who must complete items in this record have done so. Most items which must be completed in the medical record are the responsibility of a physician. Some physicians make it a weekly habit to visit

---

MERCY MEDICAL CENTER
4445 E. Short Street
Anywhere, CA 99999

June 5, 2XXX

John Doe, M.D.
555 S. Apple Street
Anywhere, CA 99999

Dear Doctor:

Since your last visit, additional medical records have been analyzed and added to your computer list. A copy of the list is enclosed. Please visit the HIM Department soon to complete them. They will not be considered delinquent until June 12, 2XXX.

During the last JCAHO survey, the hospital received a contingency because of delinquent medical records. The next progress report is due to the JCAHO in August. In order to maintain accreditation, we must reduce the number of delinquent records. Please do your part in reaching the goal.

If you have any questions or feel that the computer list contains errors, please contact Janet Mallory, Director, Health Information Management at 999-9999.

Sincerely yours,

James Samuels, M.D.
Chief of Staff

FIGURE 2.4 Sample of a letter used to notify physicians of need to complete delinquent medical records.

the HIM department to complete their incomplete records. But many physicians dislike doing "paperwork" and wait until the hospital notifies them that they must come into the department and complete the records (Figure 2.4).

Pulling for Physicians

The medical records/HIM clerk in the physician incomplete area pulls the records requiring completion by an individual physician and assists the physician when he or she comes in to finish the records. Once the physician has completed the records, the clerk checks to ensure that all documents have indeed been completed, that no entries requiring signature have been missed, and that all required reports have been dictated. If Dr. Janes comes in and completes his records but some of those records still require the work of Drs. Michaels and Miller, they are returned to the incomplete area.

We will now discuss some functions that may be found in the HIM department or may be located in individual departments.

CANCER REGISTRY

The **cancer registry** collects demographic, cancer identification, treatment, and follow-up data on each patient who is diagnosed with cancer. The data are used by physicians in planning and review of staging and treatment, research, end results, and continuing patient care. The hospital uses the data in planning for marketing and allocation of resources for cancer programs. In states where cancer is a reportable disease, the registry provides a mechanism for collecting the information that must be reported.

Cancer registries may be accredited by the American College of Surgeons (ACoS). Data collected by an accredited registry are reported to the National Cancer Data Base (NCDB). The NCDB uses the data to compare treatment and outcomes by state and nationally.

Follow-Up

Cancer registries are required to track 90 percent of their patients annually for life. That means that the registrar must annually obtain follow-up information on 90 percent of the patients in the registry. In order to do this, he or she must contact physician offices, other hospitals and healthcare facilities, and the patient's family and friends to determine where the patient has been treated, what he or she has been treated for, if the tumor has recurred, or if the patient has died.

Credentials

The National Cancer Registrar Association (NCRA) offers a Certified Tumor Registrar (CTR) credential. RHITs and RHIAs must work in a registry for twelve months prior to writing the examination. Noncredentialed staff must work in a registry two years prior to writing the examination. The ACoS encourages all registry staff to become CTRs.

Annual Report

In order to fulfill the requirements of the ACoS, the registry must publish an annual report that summarizes the activities of the cancer program during the previous calendar year. The annual report also documents the program's annual in-depth study of a cancer site, such as breast. The study includes articles about diagnosing and treating the cancer, and specific resources and support groups that address the disease process for patients and their families, written by physicians and staff at the hospital. In addition to the in-depth study, the annual report includes a statistical review of all cancer sites recorded during the previous calendar year, as well as follow-up and survival statistics.

$\mathcal{M}$EDICAL LIBRARY

The medical library consists of reference books, covering the diagnosis and treatment of different diseases, and **periodicals** from different medical associations throughout the world. Examples are the *Journal of the American Medical Association* (*JAMA*) and the *New England Journal of Medicine*. In a large facility, the medical library is usually a separate department staffed full time with a medical librarian. In a smaller hospital, the medical librarian is usually a consultant who visits the library several times a month to catalog new arrivals of periodicals and books and to make recommendations to the medical staff for the purchase of new books and educational materials. In either case, the medical librarian provides research services to any medical staff member or hospital employee who may need those services. In a small facility, the health information management director may be responsible for ensuring that the medical librarian is carrying out all functions as required by the JCAHO and the terms of the consultant's contract.

$\mathcal{C}$ASE MANAGEMENT

Case management is a process done to insure that a patient's hospital stay and services rendered are appropriate and timely. The case manager reviews the record of a current inpatient to insure that the severity of illness and/or the intensity of services being rendered meets the criteria for acute care. If not, the case manager will discuss, with the attending physician, alternatives to acute hospital care. Case managers work with all of the patient's caregivers, such as nurses, pharmacists, therapists, and so forth to insure that appropriate discharge planning occurs and that delay in conducting tests, treatments, or education does not occur.

Most insurance companies require periodic telephonic or fax notification of the case manager's review before authorizing continued hospital stay or payment of the bill. Case management helps protect the hospital, physician, and patient from denials of payment.

$\mathcal{P}$ERFORMANCE IMPROVEMENT

Performance improvement is a requirement of the JCAHO to ensure that all aspects of a hospital's performance are evaluated and improved on a continuous basis. Performance improvement teams evaluate such things as patient care, hospital environment, patient education, hospital technology, management and security of information, and safety, to name a few. During the performance improvement process, data are collected, evaluated, and benchmarked with the performance of other hospitals. Results are usually reported to a steering committee that decides on any action to be taken. Once corrective action is taken, the process begins again, with data collection, to determine if improvement has occurred. Performance improvement involves not only evaluation of areas where problems have been identified but also a periodic evaluation of all processes in the hope of improving even more.

$\mathcal{R}$ISK MANAGEMENT

Risk management is a process of addressing the risk to which patients, visitors, hospital staff, medical staff, vendors, and others are exposed. Its goal is to protect the hospital from financial loss. Hospital risk management encompasses clinical risk management, safety, and security.

Clinical risk management addresses the risks associated with patient care. Each department must have a mechanism for evaluating the risks to which patients are exposed as a result of the care and treatment received in the department and recommend methods for minimizing those risks.

The safety aspect of risk management addresses all statutes and regulations, such as building and safety codes. This includes patient and visitor safety as well as the safe working environment for the hospital and medical staff. The risk management department provides information to departments to assist in meeting requirements and monitoring compliance.

Risk management includes security for patients, visitors, staff, and hospital property, including the medical record and other confidential documents. The risk management department is instrumental in developing processes that provide for appropriate protection.

The risk manager is the recipient of all incident reports. He or she works with the hospital insurance company and/or attorney when claims or suits are submitted.

$\mathcal{S}$UMMARY

The functions performed in the health information management department affect patient care as well as hospital reimbursement. Many responsibilities require knowledge of state, federal, and other regulatory agencies. The more detailed functions, such as coding and performance improvement, require that the medical records/ HIM clerk be accurate and efficient.

$\mathcal{L}$EARNING ACTIVITIES

1. Describe the different purposes for maintaining a medical record.

2. Discuss the importance of accurate record storage and retrieval.

3. Discuss the relationship of confidentiality to the medical record.

4. What are case management, performance improvement, and risk management, and why are they important?

5. Match the definition with the correct function.

    __ **(a)** Improvement of services   **(1)** Cancer registry

    __ **(b)** Efficient use of services   **(2)** Medical transcription

    __ **(c)** Words onto paper   **(3)** Performance improvement

    __ **(d)** Classification of diseases   **(4)** Coding

    __ **(e)** Follow-up of cancer patients   **(5)** Case management

    __ **(f)** Confidentiality and patient care   **(6)** Storage and retrieval

    __ **(g)** Physician documentation   **(7)** Incomplete area

    __ **(h)** Response to requests for records   **(8)** Release of information

    __ **(i)** Reduce liability   **(9)** Risk management

Numbering and Filing Methods

VOCABULARY

Batch filing	Filing specific types of records (e.g., Emergency Department) in a pocket folder, by terminal digit.
Color coding	Assignment of a color to each digit of a medical record number.
Drop filing	Placing loose documents into the medical record file folder without fastening them into the proper area of the record.
File guide	Guides placed into the files to show where the terminal and secondary digits start.
Episode of care	Each separate occurrence in which the patient receives hospital care.
Master patient index	An index of all patients ever treated at a healthcare facility.
Middle digit filing	A method of filing in which the middle pair of digits, in the medical record number, are primary.
Outguide	A card or form that replaces a record removed from the files. It shows the new location of the record.
Serial-unit filing	A filing system in which the patient is assigned a new medical record number with each hospital encounter and in which old records are refiled under the new number.
Straight numeric filing	A filing system in which the records are filed sequentially, as the numbers are assigned.
Terminal digit filing	A numerical filing system used to distribute records evenly throughout the file area.
Unit record	A record containing the documentation of all encounters (inpatient, outpatient, and emergency room) with the healthcare facility for one patient.
Volume	An additional file folder created when the patient's medical record documentation exceeds the capacity of the original file folder.

OBJECTIVES

When you have completed this chapter, you will be able to:

- File alphabetically.
- Identify a record using any numeric filing method.
- File a record in permanent file.
- Identify a record using two color-coded systems.
- Explain the purpose for a unit record.

Health information management departments use several different filing methods, which will be discussed in detail. Alphabetical filing is used in the **master patient index** (MPI) and may be used for small groups of patient records. A numeric system is most often used for the filing of patient records in a hospital setting.

*A*LPHABETIC FILING

Alphabetical filing is done by looking at the sequence of the letters in the patient's last name. For example, *Able* would be filed before *Brett* because the letter "A" is sequenced before letter "B" in the alphabet.

When the first letter of the last name is the same, move to the sequence of the second letter in the name. *Able* is filed before *Achisan* because "b" comes before "c" in the alphabet. If the first two letters of the last name are the same, look at the sequence of the third letter and so on. *Abbott* is filed before *Abine*. When the last names are exactly the same, then look at the spelling of the first names. *Abbott, Linda,* is filed before *Abbott, Marshall.* If the last name and first name are the same, look at the sequence of the middle initial. *Abbott, Linda K.,* is filed before *Abbott, Linda M.*

Names with Prefixes

A name such as *St. John* is filed phonetically, as though it were spelled *Saint John*. Names beginning with "Mc" can be filed in a separate section alphabetically or in the "Ms" between "Ma" and "Me." Names with prefixes such as *O'Malley* or *de la Pena* are filed as though they were all one word, *Omalley* or *Delapena*.

Religious Titles

Names with religious titles, such as Sister, Father, or Reverend, should be filed using the person's last name first, and then by the religious title. Father John Fitzgerald would be filed under *Fitzgerald, Father John*.

*N*UMERIC FILING

Numeric filing utilizes a number assigned to the patient's medical record. Many hospitals use a 6-digit number divided into 3 sections of 2 digits. The numbers usually start at 00-00-01 and continue to 99-99-99, allowing most hospitals an adequate supply of numbers for many years. Hospitals with a large patient volume or that have been in business for many years may need to use a system that uses more digits. The Department of Veterans Affairs and other government hospitals use the patient's Social Security Number (123-45-6789).

Straight Numeric Filing

The most simple form of numeric filing is called **straight numeric.** Each record is assigned a number and is filed sequentially depending on the number assigned. The numbers start with 01 and continue upward. The sequence of records in a straight numeric file would be as follows:

Terminal Digit				
04	–	87	–	23
tertiary		secondary		primary
Middle Digit				
04	–	89	–	23
secondary		primary		tertiary

FIGURE 3.1 Sequence of digits in terminal digit and middle digit filing.

101	47	998
102	48	999
103	49	1,000

$\mathcal{T}$ ERMINAL DIGIT FILING

In **terminal digit filing** (Figure 3.1) the three sections from left to right are called the tertiary, secondary, and primary digits, respectively.

04	—	87	—	23
tertiary		secondary		primary

In terminal digit filing, the files are divided into 100 primary sections, starting with 00 and ending with 99. To file a record, first go to the file section corresponding to the primary digits in the patient's number. In that section look for a subsection matching the secondary digits in the number. Then file the record numerically according to the tertiary digits. The sequence of records in the file is as follows:

04-87-23	97-11-34	98-99-68
05-87-23	98-11-34	99-99-68
06-87-23	99-11-34	00-00-69
07-87-23	00-12-34	01-00-69

Advantages

The advantages to terminal digit filing over straight numerical filing is that the files are distributed evenly because records will go into each of the 100 primary digit sections before repeating. In a straight numerical system (i.e., 00-00-69, 00-00-70, 00-00-71) the newest records are all filed in one section of the files; file space is rapidly depleted and records must be shifted often.

$\mathcal{M}$ IDDLE DIGIT FILING

Middle digit filing uses the same six-digit, three-section numbers as terminal digit filing. The difference is in the primary, secondary, and tertiary positions. The middle pair of digits is primary, the left pair is secondary, and the right pair is tertiary.

04	—	89	—	23
secondary		primary		tertiary

The sequence of records in the file is as follows:

04-89-23	05-98-12	98-98-98
04-89-24	05-98-13	98-98-99
04-89-25	05-98-14	98-99-00
04-89-26	05-98-15	98-99-01

Middle digit filing also provides for more even distribution of records than straight numerical filing.

Another Numeric Filing Method

Another filing method is to have the digits secondary, tertiary, primary from left to right.

02	—	75	—	33
secondary		tertiary		primary

The file sequence is as follows:

02-75-33	06-98-24
02-76-33	06-99-24
02-77-33	07-00-24
02-78-33	07-01-24

𝒰NIT AND SERIAL NUMBERING

Unit Numbering

In this system, the patient is assigned a medical record number on the first encounter with the hospital. Any subsequent encounters will be identified with the same number. Because the same number is used, all documents are automatically filed in one location.

Serial Numbering

In a **serial unit** system, the patient is assigned a different medical record number for each **episode of care** at the hospital. Multiple records for the same patient will be stored in different locations.

Creating a Unit Record

A **unit record** means all documents pertaining to a patient's encounters at a hospital are filed in one location or portions of the record filed in separate areas can be easily retrieved as needed for patient care. The JCAHO prefers the unit record because all information about a patient is readily available. Using a unit number automatically creates a unit record because all documents will be identified with the same number. With serial numbering, a unit record is created by pulling forward records filed under the old number assigned to the patient and refiling them under the number being used to identify the information for the patient's current visit. An incomplete record could result if all previous information is not pulled forward. If there is a large readmission rate, the medical records/HIM clerk spends much more time refiling records.

File Guides

File guides may be used by a health information management department to increase the ease and speed of filing and retrieving records. These guides are placed at the beginning of number sections. The frequency of guides will probably increase as the activity of the files increases. The guides are usually made of a durable material with a tab that sticks out beyond the edges of the file folders. The guides for the terminal digit 23 would appear as follows:

<u>00</u>   <u>01</u>   <u>02</u>
23   23   23

The top set of digits refers to the secondary digits. The first record to be found after the guide 02/23 would be 00-02-23, followed by 01-02-23, and so on.

COLOR CODING

In order to reduce the number of misfiles and facilitate retrieval of a record, most HIM departments use **color coding** on their file folders. Each number from 0 to 9 is assigned a color. Color bars are placed on the edge of the file folder to correspond with the medical record number. Usually only the primary digits are color coded, for simplicity; however, some departments use color coding for three, four, or more digits. When records are filed in correct numerical sequence, the color bands create a distinct color pattern (Figure 3.2). Misfiles are easily identified. Also, records not yet filed can be more readily identified by looking for the correct color bars.

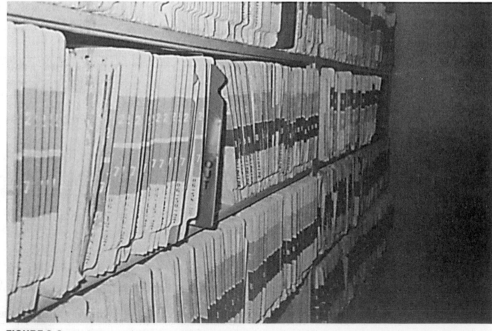

FIGURE 3.2 The color codes create a distinct pattern.

Standard Color-Coding Systems

There are two standard color-coding systems. Ames Color File manufactures file folders using the following colors:

0—red	1—gray	2—blue
3—orange	4—purple	5—black
6—yellow	7—brown	8—pink
9—green		

Smead Corporation uses the following designation:

0—yellow	1—blue	2—pink
3—purple	4—orange	5—brown
6—green	7—gray	8—red
9—black		

Please note that your department may use a unique color-coding system.

*O*UTGUIDES

Outguides are used in some health information management departments to indicate that a record has been removed from the files. Outguides (Figure 3.3) are made of a durable material such as plastic and contain one or two pockets to hold loose

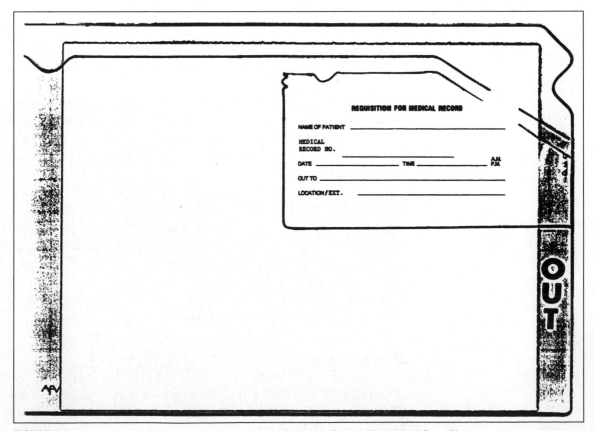

FIGURE 3.3 An example of an outguide used to mark the location of a record removed from file.

documents or record requisitions. Departments with a high retrieval volume may use a different color outguide for each day of the week. This procedure facilitates identifying those records that have been out of file longer than department policy permits.

FILING LOOSE DOCUMENTS

All health information management departments receive loose documents daily, which must be filed in the appropriate medical records. Loose documents consist of test results for patients who have left the facility or dictated reports, such as consultation and operative reports. Because these documents can affect patient care and hospital reimbursement, they should be filed as soon as possible. If the record cannot be located, the document may be placed in an outguide, which is then filed in the space where the record should be. Before filing any record in the permanent file, all loose documents should be filed into the record securely. Because a unit record contains all treatment episodes, it is important to match the date of the document with the correct episode of care. Placing a document in the wrong episode of care is almost the same as throwing the document away.

Drop Filing

In departments with a high volume of emergency and diagnostic patients, the amount of loose filing received daily may overwhelm the resources of HIM. Rather than having stacks of documents pile up, the department may decide to **drop file.** This means that the documents are placed in the file folder without being fastened down. HIM will usually have a policy that the documents are secured into the correct episode of care at the time the record is next pulled for a requestor.

Fasteners

Documents are kept secure in a medical record with the use of a fastener in the file folder. These fasteners usually are preapplied to the folder, but self-adhesive types are available. Depending on the design of the medical record forms and inpatient chart holders in the hospital, the fasteners may be located at the top or on the side of the folder. Every HIM department has a different configuration of the documents in the file folder. For example, inpatient records may be filed on the right side of the folder, and outpatient, emergency department, and other miscellaneous records may be filed on the left side of the folder.

Hole Punching

Most medical record forms are prepunched with the correct number and placement of holes to fit over the rings in the nursing station binder and the fastener in the medical record file folder. If manually punching holes in a document, the medical records/HIM clerk should be careful that the paper is placed completely into the punch. This ensures that the holes are not on the edge of the form, resulting in tears. There are commercial products available for reinforcing holes.

VOLUMES

The majority of medical record file folders are designed to hold approximately 2 inches of documentation. More than that causes the folder to close improperly, leading to torn documents. Whenever a record's size exceeds that of its file folder, it should be broken down into another **volume.** To differentiate between the volumes, they should be labeled 1 of 2 and 2 of 2. If additional volumes are created, the previous volumes' labeling should be changed to reflect the current number of volumes. The volumes become 1 of 3, 2 of 3, 3 of 3, and so on. The oldest records should start in Volume 1 and continue chronologically through the most current volume.

When a patient's stay in the hospital is so long that the record will not fit into a single file folder, it is necessary to break the episode of care into two or more file folders. In this case the folders are labeled Volume 1 with additional labels such as Part A, Part B, and so forth.

*S*TEP-BY-STEP PROCEDURE FOR FILING A RECORD USING TERMINAL DIGIT FILING

1. If the record is too large for the file folder, break it down into volumes.

2. Repair any torn pages.

3. Identify the primary digits.

4. Go to the area of files corresponding with primary digits.

5. Look for the file guide corresponding to the secondary and primary digits or look for color bars corresponding to primary digits.

6. If the hospital uses outguides, pull the outguide from the files. Fasten down any loose documents found in the outguide in the correct chart order under the correct episode of care (see Chapter 5).

7. File the record in the correct sequence according to the tertiary digits.

If the record cannot easily be pushed into its correct location, do not force it. The files may have to be adjusted to make room for the record. There should be enough room so that each record fits into the shelf properly and the different records side by side create a straight line. Records that are forced into a space that is too small will tear and look disorderly (Figure 3.4).

Health information management departments have an ongoing issue with storage space for medical record filing. To free space in the files, most departments periodically purge inactive records. The purged records may be stored in boxes or open shelving in a different location on the hospital grounds. More likely, they are sent to a contract storage company that provides retrieval services. Other alternatives include converting to microfilm or optical imaging.

Records to be purged are usually selected based on the amount of file space available and the last date of treatment. If the department has room to store only two years of records, the record of any patient whose last date of treatment was more than two years ago will be pulled out. The advantage to this system is that the entire record is stored in one place. The year grid or label on the file folder helps the clerk identify the last year of treatment. The hospital computer system may be able to produce a list of records meeting the purge criteria. Some hospitals go through each record on the shelf and pull out the documentation that is older than the retention period. In hospitals with a stable patient population who return frequently, more space is freed in the files by using this method.

The permanent retention of records can be quite costly. Storage facilities charge for retrieval and refiling, as well as permanent removal. Some states have statutes that specify the length of retention. In California, the record must be kept seven years past the last date of treatment, unless the patient is a minor. Minors' records must be

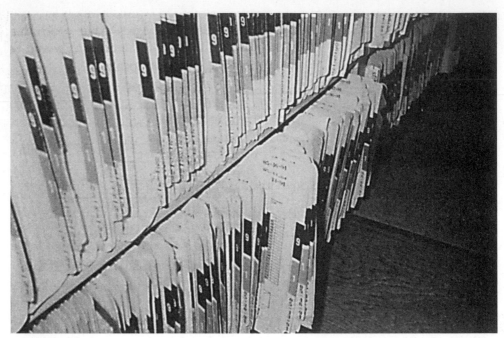

FIGURE 3.4 Records shoved in inadequate space stick out in a disorderly fashion.

kept seven years or until age 19, whichever is greater. Another exception are newborn records. Both the baby's and the mother's delivery record, including fetal monitor strips, must be kept until age 19. Other states, such as Wisconsin, have no statute specifying how long records must be maintained.

B ATCH FILING

Another method that can save space and time is **batch filing.** In batch filing each terminal digit has a color-coded pocket folder that is filed at the beginning of each terminal digit in the file area. The records of patients who are treated only in the Emergency Department or for diagnostic tests are filed in terminal digit order within the batch folders. This saves the time and cost of making individual file folders for these patients and meets the definition of a unit record, as a patient's batch records can easily be pulled as needed. Usually, when a patient is admitted as an inpatient or for outpatient surgery, any batch records for that patient are pulled from the batch folder and filed into the individual file folder. If a patient accumulates five batch records, they will be pulled from the batch folder and a file folder will be created for the patient.

S UMMARY

The health information management department uses both alphabetical and numeric filing systems to identify patient information and records. The ability to file and retrieve a medical record correctly is one of the most important tasks a medical record clerk must learn. A number of systems, including color coding, outguides, and fasteners, aids the efficiency of the filing function.

LEARNING ACTIVITIES

1. Place the following names in alphabetical order.

   Jones, Gerald A.   Richards, Kathleen P.
   Richards, Kathleen L.   Richards, Peter T.
   Jons, James O.   O'Brian, John B.
   Reiger, Karen C.   Rieger, Karen D.
   O'Brien, Sister Mary Agnes

2. Place the following medical record numbers in straight numerical order, terminal digit order, and middle digit order.

00-14-86	22-01-00	11-15-66
00-15-87	10-15-66	10-16-66
21-12-99	00-15-86	22-99-00
21-15-99	00-17-86	11-14-67

3. Using a terminal digit system, relate the steps in locating the following records in permanent file.

06-34-15	13-99-62
02-99-37	99-48-00

4. Using the Smead and Ames color codes, respectively, and using terminal digit filing, fill in the two colors that would be on the file folders of the following medical records numbers.

Smead			**Ames**	
00-16-34	____	____	____	____
06-98-57	____	____	____	____
14-31-82	____	____	____	____
14-75-14	____	____	____	____
03-03-03	____	____	____	____
00-12-00	____	____	____	____
23-44-46	____	____	____	____
75-57-75	____	____	____	____
09-80-66	____	____	____	____
12-24-48	____	____	____	____

5. Repeat Exercise 4, using middle digit filing.

6. Discuss the two methods of purging records and the advantages and disadvantages of each.

7. Define drop filing and explain its advantages and disadvantages.

8. Explain when batch filing is used and why.

## CHAPTER 4

Processing Medical Records

Imprinter plate A plastic plate, similar to a charge card, on which identifying information, such as the patient's name, age, account number, and medical record number, are embossed. The embossed card is then used in a machine with ink to imprint the information from the card onto each document in the patient's record.

Permanent file The file area for records whose documentation is complete.

Preadmission Collection of patient demographic and insurance information prior to the patient's admission.

Record retrieval Identifying the location of a record and pulling from the files.

Requisition A document used in an outguide to identify the record that has been pulled.

Thinned record Removal of the oldest portions of a record from the nursing unit binder when the record becomes too large for the binder.

Temporary folder A file folder created to house an incomplete medical record until it is ready to be filed in the original folder.

When you have completed this chapter, you will be able to:

- Explain the purpose for the master patient index and be able to update it either manually or on a computer.
- Correct master patient index errors.
- Process admissions and discharges.
- Pull lists efficiently and check out records.

MASTER PATIENT INDEX

The master patient index (MPI) is the record of all patients treated for any reason at the hospital. It is the only place to look up a patient by name to retrieve the medical record number. The MPI also lists all visits for each patient. Because of its importance in identifying patients, it should never be destroyed.

The importance of accuracy in maintaining the MPI cannot be overemphasized. If the patient's medical record number is recorded incorrectly, the department may never be able to locate the record. If the name is recorded incorrectly, the department may tell a requester that it has no record, when, in fact, one does exist.

```
332456              MR05-32-98        678 Apple Lane
ADAMS, EDITH P.                       Anywhere, CA  99999
Dr. G. Hall                           999-9999
DOB 12-23-1965
─────────────────────────────────────────────────────────
Admitted:  6/5/2XXX OPS
Admitted:  5/30/2XXX             Disch:  JUN 0 2 2XXX
```

FIGURE 4.1 An example of a manual master patient index (MPI) card.

Manual MPI

The MPI can be maintained manually or on a computer. A manual MPI is usually maintained on 3″ × 5″ index cards (Figure 4.1). When a person first becomes a patient, his or her name is typed or imprinted on the card, along with the date of birth. The cards may be generated by the admitting department. Cards may have headings for admission and discharge dates, type of service (for example, inpatient, outpatient, or emergency department), and attending physician. The amount of information is limited by the size of the card and may vary by hospital. The MPI is updated whenever the patient receives additional treatment. The new treatment dates are added along with the other information required on the card. Some hospitals update the patient's address on the MPI card; others do so only in the actual medical record. Correct updating of the MPI card is important so that all episodes of care can be identified and filed in the unit medical record.

Assignment of Medical Record Number

Medical record numbers are usually assigned by the admitting department from a list of unused numbers, when there is no computer system. In a unit record system, admitting must check the MPI to determine if the patient has been treated before. If the patient has been seen before, the admitting clerk will obtain the previous medical record number for the current episode of care. If no previous records exist, a new number will be assigned. If the check is done carelessly or not at all, a patient may be assigned a second medical record number in error (Figure 4.2).

$\mathcal{M}$ASTER PATIENT INDEX FILE ERRORS

Occasionally, when you are filing new MPI cards, you may discover that an MPI card has been created for a patient who already has a card in the index. Check the cards carefully to ensure that they are actually the same patient. The birth dates should be

```
344879                    MR05-31-11        232 South St.
JONES, FRANK K.                             Anywhere, CA  99999
Dr. S. Johnson                              999-9999
DOB 5/6/1943
────────────────────────────────────────────────────────────────
Admit:  10/22/2XXX          Disch:
Admit:   8/16/2XXX    OPS          OCT 27 2XXX
```

```
444776                    MR06-40-50        232 South St.
JONES, FRANK K.                             Anywhere, CA 99999
Dr. S. Johnson                              999-9999
DOB 5/6/1943
────────────────────────────────────────────────────────────────
Admit:    5/15/2XXX         Disch:
                                   MAY 25 2XXX
```

FIGURE 4.2 Patient assigned two medical record numbers. Top card is the old MPI entry. Bottom card reveals a second number.

the same. You may find that everything matches except that one patient has a middle initial and the other does not. In a small facility, a probable assumption is that the two cards belong to the same patient. In a large facility, however, such an assumption should never be made. The greater the number of patients, the greater the chance that two different patients with the same name and birth date could be admitted. The only totally accurate way to determine if the cards belong to two separate patients is to pull the records and see if there are similarities.

One Patient with Two Medical Record Numbers

Select one number as the file number for the patient's record. Depending on the health information management department policy, this may be the old number, not the new number. If the new number is selected, bring all previous documents forward to the new number. If the old number is selected, renumber the current documents and file them under the old number. Correct the MPI to reflect the number selected. Cross-reference the discarded number to the selected number. Do not allow the discarded number to be reissued to another patient.

Two Patients with the Same Medical Record Number

Another error that can occur is two patients being assigned the same medical record number.

New Patients with Different Names.   If both are new patients and have different names, correct the error as follows:

1. The second patient to receive the number must be assigned a new medical record number from the log.

2. If the patient is in-house, a new **imprinter plate** must be made for that patient and sent to the nursing station.

3. In the HIM department, the MPI card must be corrected to show the newly assigned medical record number. Process a new file folder.

4. Separate documents if interfiling of both patients' records occurred.

Two Patients with the Same Name.   If the two patients with the same name are assigned to one number, correct the error as follows:

1. The second patient to receive the number must be given a new medical record number.

2. Change the MPI cards for both patients.
   a. First patient: Remove the visit data that belong to the second patient.
   b. Second patient: Create a new card.

3. If the second patient is in-house, a new imprinter card must be made for that patient and sent to the nursing station.

4. If the first patient's records were brought forward, they must be returned to the original file.

5. If the second patient's records were interfiled with the first patient's, remove the second patient's records and file under the new medical record number.

Two MPI Cards Belonging to One Patient

If you determine that the two cards belong to the same patient, the following action must occur:

1. If the medical record numbers are the same, transfer the most recent information to the first card generated.

2. Destroy the second card.

3. If the medical record numbers are not the same, follow the procedures under One Patient with Two Medical Record Numbers.

COMPUTERIZED MASTER PATIENT INDEXES

Most hospitals have computerized MPIs. There are many advantages to this type of system over a manual MPI. The amount of data that can be maintained on each patient is greater. Updating information is faster and easier. The health information management department no longer needs to make space for a rotary or stacked card file.

The disadvantage to computerized systems is that errors may not be as easily corrected as in a manual system.

Assignment of Medical Record Number

On a computerized MPI, the admitting clerk no longer assigns the medical record number from a list. When all information required to admit a patient has been entered, the computer automatically assigns the next number. The computer relies on the information entered to reach its conclusions; if the admitting clerk does not enter the patient's name exactly as it was entered previously, the computer may erroneously show that the patient has no existing number and will assign a new medical record number.

Searching for Patient Name

To avoid such errors, the clerk should conduct a partial search by entering a few letters of the patient's last name and a designated symbol, such as an asterisk. Some computer systems will conduct a partial search without a symbol. The symbol tells the computer to search for all names that begin with those letters. The computer will then provide a list of all patients previously treated, whose last names begin with the same letters. The clerk can then search the list and pick out the patient, verifying name and birth date. For example, if the clerk is looking for Mary B. Benton, he or she would type in BEN*. Without the symbol, the computer would look only for the name "BEN." The list provided might look like this:

NAME	DOB
BENATTON, GEORGE N.	10/02/1943
BENSON, JULIE T.	05/06/1961
BENTON, MARY A.	04/30/1956
BENTON, MARY B.	12/02/1954

This same procedure should be followed by the medical records/HIM clerk checking the MPI for the medical record number or previous dates of treatment.

Error Correction

The same types of errors that can be made in a manual MPI can also be made in a computer system. Correction of those errors in a computer system can be more time-consuming and, depending on the software, may be extremely difficult.

One Patient with Two Numbers

If a patient is erroneously assigned two medical record numbers, one of the numbers (usually the one assigned second) must be deleted for that patient. As in the manual system, the patient information listed under the erroneous medical record number must be transferred to the selected number prior to deleting the erroneous number.

```
                                        HSP M.P.I.  (DEMOG/VISIT) INQUIRY
                                                   ENTER LINE # -----
LN    PATIENT NAME          SEX        DOB         ADDRESS          MED.REC. #
01    HITCHCOCK, JANICE     F          04/16/1988  669 ELM ST          34567
02    HITCHCOCK, JANICE     F          04/16/1988  669 ELM ST          56789
03
04
```

MPI inquiry shows that patient Janet Hitchcock has two medical record numbers.

```
                                        HSP M.P.I. (DEMOG/VISIT) INQUIRY
                                                   ENTER LINE # -----
MED.REC. #:   34567         PATIENT NAME:   HITCHCOCK, JANICE
LN    ACCT. #           ADMIT DT    DISCH DT    PTP
01    123321            03/07/2008  03/11/2008  INP
02
03
04
```

Visit inquiry for first number shows one account number.

```
                                        HSP M.P.I. (DEMOG/VISIT) INQUIRY
                                                   ENTER LINE # -----
MED.REC. #:   56789         PATIENT NAME:   HITCHCOCK, JANICE
LN    ACCT. #           ADMIT DT    DISCH DT    PTP
01    918257            04/26/2009  05/01/2009  INP
02
03
04
```

Visit inquiry for second number shows one account number.

```
                                        HSP M.P.I. (DEMOG/VISIT) INQUIRY
                                                   ENTER LINE # -----
MED.REC. #:   34567         PATIENT NAME:   HITCHCOCK, JANICE
LN    ACCT. #           ADMIT DT    DISCH DT    PTP
01    123321            03/07/2008  03/11/2008  INP
02    918257            04/26/2009  05/01/2009  INP
03
04
```

Account number 918257 has been moved from medical record number 56789 to medical record number 34567.

FIGURE 4.3 Computer MPI screens showing a patient with two medical record numbers and the correction of an error.

Depending on the computer system, this might be done by transferring the patient account number (billing number) from the second medical record number to the first (Figure 4.3). When this occurs, all of the demographic information associated with that account number will also be transferred to the first medical record number. If no patient information is associated with the erroneous medical record number, it can be deleted.

Two Patients with the Same Number

Another error that can occur is two patients being assigned the same medical record number. This occurs when the admitting clerk fails to check the MPI properly to ascertain that a patient does or does not have an existing medical record number. In this situation, the second patient assigned the number must be assigned a new, unique medical record number. Usually medical record numbers are assigned automatically only when a patient is being admitted or registered for some type of treatment. In the case where the patient has been assigned the wrong medical record number, the demographic data is already in the system. If the patient were admitted or registered with a new number and the same demographic data, a duplicate entry would result. Depending on the capabilities of the computer system, it may be necessary to "preadmit" the patient in order for the system to assign a new medical and insurance information record number to that patient. **Preadmission** is the collection of demographic data prior to the patient's admission. The account number and demographic data pertaining to the visit may be moved from the patient index entry with the wrong medical record number to the newly created one. The preadmission for that patient is then cancelled. The result of this process is that the patient has been assigned his or her own unique medical record number; the demographic information for the patient's hospitalization has been moved to that number; and no additional erroneous information has been added to the MPI. The methods for merging duplicate numbers will vary based on the computer system used.

$\mathcal{A}$DMISSION PROCESSING

The health information management department does not receive the medical record until the patient's encounter with the hospital (i.e., inpatient, outpatient, emergency room treatment) has been completed. However, the department may process admissions and registrations on a daily basis. This might be done so the department is ready to receive the record and to identify any errors that may have occurred. In order to save staff time, many departments conduct all processing at discharge.

Procedure for Processing Admissions

An HIM department procedure for processing admissions might be as follows:

1. Pick up medical record copies of patient registration forms from admitting.

2. Verify that you have received all registration forms by checking them against the list of admissions and registrations for the previous day. This list may be generated by the admitting department or by a computer system. If there is a discrepancy, check with the statistician in the HIM department who has the nursing floor census sheets for the previous day.

3. Check the MPI to verify that the patient's name is spelled correctly and to ensure that a duplicate medical record number has not been assigned.
   a. If an error has been made, take the necessary steps to make corrections.
   b. Notify admitting so that a new imprinter plate can be made with the correct information for the patient.

4. If using a manual MPI, remove the index card and place an "Out" card in its place.

5. Type the admit or visit date on the MPI card. (This step will be omitted if there is a computer system. With a computerized MPI, the visit information is updated through the admitting process.)

6. Make a file folder for each patient.
   a. New patients
      (1) Pull a blank folder corresponding to the assigned medical record number or to the terminal digit color codes (Figure 4.4).
      (2) Print the patient's name in the designated area of the file folder in the format of last name, first name, and middle initial.

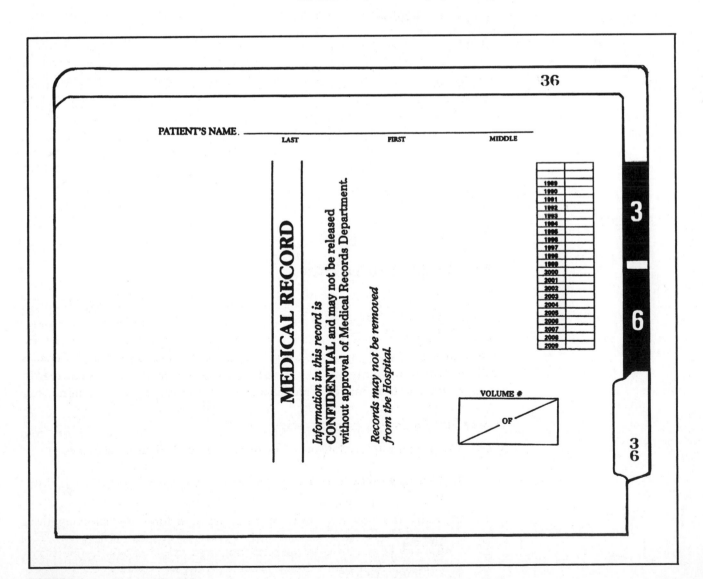

FIGURE 4.4 A color-coded file folder.

(3) Mark the current year on the year-of-service grid, if there is no year label.

b. Readmitted patients—Pull the old record from the files.

7. File all in-house folders together in alphabetical or terminal digit order.

8. File registration forms alphabetically in the in-house box or with the file folders.

9. File MPI cards alphabetically in the in-house box or with the file folders.

10. Pull any previous records and deliver to the nursing station.

In the preceding procedure, registration forms are filed in a box for ease in providing information and copies to physician offices and other requesters as requested. MPI cards are filed separately to ensure that the discharge date is entered when the patient has been discharged. In a computer system, there will be no MPI cards to file or registration forms to pick up and file. A list of admissions and discharges will be generated by the system daily.

Temporary Folder

A **temporary folder** may be used for a readmitted patient to facilitate completion of the record and to reduce the amount of space necessary for filing incomplete records. If a patient has many encounters with the facility, the record can be large. Large records take up more space and are more difficult to use. Also, if the patient has been recently discharged and then readmitted, there will be two incomplete records. Filing them on top of each other can increase the likelihood of a physician becoming confused and failing to complete all items in the record. At many hospitals all records are filed in the permanent folder at discharge, no matter how many incomplete episodes of care there are. When using temporary records, each individual hospitalization is filed in the permanent file folder only when it is complete.

*D*ISCHARGE PROCESSING

Procedure for Processing Discharges

Once a patient admission or visit has ended, the majority of the medical record clerk's work begins. The following is a procedure that might be used to process records of discharged patients:

1. Pick up discharge records from each nursing station. Pick up visit records from clinics, the emergency room, outpatient surgery, and other departments. Note that in some facilities the treating area, such as the nursing unit or clinic, may deliver records to the HIM department.

2. Verify correct number of records and names with the discharge list from the admitting department, the computer-generated discharge list, or the registration list.

3. Pull registration forms, MPI cards, and file folders from their respective in-house sections, if admission processing is done.

4. Stamp the discharge date on the original registration form in the record, the registration form copy, and the MPI card. This step is necessary only for inpatients. Stamping the MPI card is not necessary if the hospital has a computerized MPI.

5. Place each record in its folder.

6. Count folders and registration forms and verify that all records have been picked up. Notify your supervisor and the nursing supervisor of any missing records.

7. File registration forms in current month folder.

8. File back MPI cards alphabetically in the MPI. (This step is not necessary with a computerized MPI.)

9. Attach loose documents to the records.

10. File records in alphabetical order or terminal digit order behind the file guide pertaining to the discharge date, in the "Records to Be Coded" section.

Filing Registration Forms

The filing of registration forms, in Step 7, is done for speed and efficiency in hospitals without computer systems that allow reprinting of registration sheets. The health information management department receives numerous requests for patient information and/or copies of registration forms from physician offices. Having the forms filed alphabetically by month allows the retrieval of the necessary information quickly and without having to locate and disassemble the actual medical record.

Serial-Unit Records

In a hospital using a serial-unit system, the old records will be pulled forward and given the new number when the patient is discharged.

Assembly

In some health information management departments, the medical records/HIM clerk may be required to add a step between Steps 9 and 10. Assembly of the record, which will be discussed in Chapter 5, may be conducted prior to coding the record. Depending on the volume of discharges and the staffing of the department, the medical records/HIM clerk processing discharges may also assemble the records.

Thinned Records

While a patient is an inpatient, the medical record is kept in a binder on the nursing station. If the patient's length of stay is long, the binder may become too full to add additional documents. To make room, the record is thinned. This means that the oldest forms, progress notes and orders, for example, with voluminous documentation are removed from the binder and secured with a fastener such as a rubber band. Usually, the dictated reports and face sheet will remain in the binder. The **thinned records** may be kept on the nursing station or in the HIM department until the patient is discharged and the record assembled. If the patient is an inpatient for many weeks, there may be more than one set of thinned documents.

Processing Outpatient Records—Alternative Method

Because most outpatients stay in the hospital less than 24 hours, the file folder can be created at the time the record is received in the department rather than at the time of admission. The documents in an outpatient record, including emergency room visits, may be filed on the left side of the file folder so as to remain separate from the inpatient admissions. As with inpatient records, it is important to check for loose documents when assembling the record prior to coding.

Referred Outpatient Records

A patient who is sent by his or her physician to the hospital for a test or treatment is known as a referred patient. These tests or treatments might include visits to the laboratory, radiology, respiratory therapy, cardiac rehabilitation, or physical therapy. The HIM department may be responsible for filing the records of referred outpatients. However, some departments, such as the laboratory and respiratory therapy, may be required by state law to keep their own copies of test results.

$\mathcal{R}$ ECORD RETRIEVAL

Retrieval of records from lists submitted by individual requesters can be a major function of a medical records/HIM clerk. Most HIM departments have policies regarding the lists that are submitted to the department. The more information that the requester can provide about a particular record, the easier it is to retrieve. Usually, the minimal information acceptable on a list is the patient's name and the date of treatment. If the requester has access to the medical record number, it should also be included on the list. However, as a medical records/HIM clerk, you may be required to look up patient names in the MPI in order to determine the medical record numbers under which records are located.

Requisitions

Once you have identified the medical record numbers for all patients on the list, you are ready to pull the records. If your department uses a manual **outguide** system, you will need to prepare a **requisition** (Figure 4.5) for each record on the list. A requisition is a document that lists the patient's name, medical record number, name and location of requester, and the date the record is pulled. Some hospitals use a two-part form, placing the original in the outguide and attaching the carbon to the record to remind the requester that it is checked out. If your department uses a computerized locator system for checking out records, you can stick this step. Place the requisitions in terminal digit order.

Terminal Digit Order

The objective in record retrieval is to find the records as quickly as possible while looking in the fewest possible places. If the dates of treatment requested are for patients recently discharged, the records are probably in the incomplete file area. It

```
+-----------------------------------------------------------+
|                                                           |
|          REQUISITION FOR MEDICAL RECORD                   |
|                                                           |
|   NAME OF PATIENT_____       |
|                                                           |
|   MEDICAL RECORD NO._____        |
|                                                      AM   |
|   DATE_____  TIME_____   PM   |
|                                                           |
|   OUT TO_____        |
|                                                           |
|   LOCATION/EXT._____        |
|                                                           |
+-----------------------------------------------------------+
```

FIGURE 4.5 An example of a medical record requisition.

would be a waste of time to start searching in **permanent file** for those records. By placing the requisitions or list in terminal digit order, you can start at the beginning of the files and work toward the 99s. This saves time and energy that would be spent moving repeatedly from one end of the files to the other if the requisitions were not in terminal digit order.

Retrieve Records by Section

Retrieve all the records you can find in each section. For example, look for all the records in the incomplete file area and then go to the permanent file area, rather than going back and forth. You may wish to make notes on the requisition or list the areas checked to avoid repeating a search. As you pull each record, place the requisition in an outguide and place the outguide in the file space where the record was pulled. If using a list, check off each record as it is located. If you cannot find a record, go on to the next requisition or number on the list.

Continue Search for Hard-to-Find Records

Once you have found all the records that are easily located, take the remaining requisitions and start looking for the records, one by one, in all the areas in the medical record department where records might be located. For example, a record could be on another employee's desk, or it may have been pulled and not checked out properly. If further search still produces no record, it may be misfiled.

$\mathcal{P}$ROCEDUE FOR LOCATING MISFILES

The following methods for locating a misfile are reprinted courtesy of Physicians' Record Company:

1. Look for transpositions of the last two digits of the number, or of the hundreds or thousands digits. The number 46-37-82 may be filed as 46-37-28 or 46-73-82.

2. Look for misfiles of "3" under "5" or "8" and vice versa; and of "7" or "8" under "9." The number "9" may be taken for a "7" if it is worn.

3. Check for a certain number in the hundred group just preceding or following the number, as 485 under 385 or 585, or under other similar combinations.

4. Check for transpositions of first and last numbers.

5. Check the folder just before and just after the one needed. It sometimes happens that a folder is put into another folder rather than between two folders.

Signing out Records

After locating and pulling the records on a list, using the computer system, you must then sign them out to the requestor. In some systems, you can choose the requestor from a list and then enter the medical record numbers one after the other. Other systems require that each medical record number be entered individually. Then the system will prompt you to select the episode of care or volume being checked out. The advantage of using a computer system is that anyone in need of a record can instantly see where it is checked out to instead of having to go to the file area and look for a requisition.

Signing in Records

Every record signed out must be signed back into the department after the requestor is finished with it. Again, the method for this will depend on the computer system used by your HIM department. If the record is not signed in and is placed back into the file area, you and your co-workers may spend a lot of wasted time looking for the record in the wrong place.

When refiling a record in the file area, remove the outguide and discard the requisition first. If this isn't done, the next clerk searching for the record may see the outguide with the old requisition first and waste time trying to find a record that is no longer signed out

SUMMARY

The master patient index (MPI) identifies each patient by a unique medical record number and gives information about each encounter with the hospital. The medical records/HIM clerk must be able to use and update the MPI accurately and efficiently so that medical records can be processed and retrieved on a daily basis. Each health information management department has systematic procedures for processing admissions and discharges and for pulling lists of records.

Consistently signing records out of and back into HIM is very important to the efficient operation of the department.

LEARNING ACTIVITIES

1. Jean K. Smith, DOB 6/9/1974, is admitted as an inpatient on 2/14/2005. Upon checking the computer MPI the next day, the medical records/HIM clerk finds the following entry:

NAME	SEX	DOB	MR#
Smith, Jean L.	F	05241968	064030
Smith, Jean K.	F	06091974	064030

The detail screen is as follows:

Med Rec # 064030 Patient Name: Smith, Jean L.

LN	ACCT #	ADMIT DT	DISCH DT
01	300107	05102002	05152002
02	302564	11252003	12012003
03	309487	02142005	

What is the error on these screens? What steps should be taken to correct the error? Show how the screen will look when the error is corrected.

2. Upon checking the computerized MPI, the medical records/HIM clerk finds the following entry:

NAME	SEX	DOB	MR#
Harper, Thomas E.	M	06251981	055782
Harper, Thomas E.	M	06251981	059998

The detail screens are as follows:

Med Rec # 055782 Patient Name: Harper, Thomas E.

LN	ACCT #	ADMIT DT	DISCH DT
01	280671	12122003	12142003

Med Rec # 059998 Patient Name: Harper, Thomas E.

LN	ACCT #	ADMIT DT	DISCH DT
01	280982	01232004	01262004

What is the possible error on this screen? What steps should be taken to verify that an error exists and then to correct the error? How will the detail screen look when the error is corrected?

3. The medical records/HIM clerk is filing the following index card in the MPI:

MR.05-60-46   DOB: 2/19/1943
Sullivan, James T.

ADMITTED	PAT. TYPE	DISCHARGED
7/13/2003	Inpt.	7/16/2003
8/10/2003	OPS	
9/9/2004	Inpt.	9/13/2004

In the MPI, he or she finds the following card:

MR.05-60-46   DOB: 2/19/1943
Sullivan, James T.

ADMITTED	PAT. TYPE	DISCHARGED
6/24/2002	ER	
9/6/2004	ER	

What is the error? What steps should be taken to correct the error? How should the card look after the error is corrected?

4. The following records have been searched for without success. Relate the steps in checking for a misfile for each of the following records.

04-23-39   21-18-48
10-75-97   05-44-65

5. While processing admissions, the medical records/HIM clerk notices a registration form for patient Marie Anderson, DOB 3/31/1975. The DOB and address are the same as that of Marie Andersen, on a card already filed in the MPI. What should the clerk do?

6. Using 3″ × 5″ cards, create MPI cards using the following information. File the cards in alphabetical order. Do not discard, as they will be used in Exercise 7.

Miller, David M.
MR 03-56-00
DOB 3/20/1978
Admit: 6/5/2008 OPS

Serface, Sheryl
MR 05-54-74
DOB 2/7/1968
Admit: 3/6/2007 ER
Admit: 1/30/2008 OPS
Admit: 2/5/2008
Disch.: 2/10/2008

O'Hara, Kate S.
MR 04-56-78
DOB 4/16/1966
Admit: 12/12/2007
Disch.: 12/12/2007

Burde, Peter
MR 04-45-46
DOB 5/5/1980
Admit: 8/8/2006
Disch.: 8/14/2006

Richards, Roger D.
MR 06-20-55
DOB 8/19/1943
Admit: 5/16/2006
Disch.: 5/18/2006
Admit: 4/1/2007 OPS
Admit: 8/29/2008 ER

Adams, Patrice B.
MR 04-59-17
DOB 1/1/1985
Admit: 3/3/2008 ER
Admit: 4/10/2008 ER
Admit: 5/15/2008 ER

Kirk, Thomas J.
MR 04-12-99
DOB 7/3/2000
Admit: 8/3/2000
Disch.: 8/5/2000

Jordan, Richard
MR 04-46-23
DOB 9/11/1933
Admit: 3/4/2005
Disch.: 3/21/2005
Admit: 5/1/2007 OPS
Admit 3/4/2009
Disch.: 3/6/2009

7. The following is the admission and discharge list for Mercy Hospital for a three-day period. Use the MPI created in Exercise 6 as the existing hospital MPI. As the medical records/HIM clerk, process the admissions and discharges. Assume that the file folders for patients discharged on 5/10/2010 were created upon admission. Use manila folders and 3″ × 5″ index cards to create file folders and new MPI cards. Use either the Ames or Smead color codes; if colored tape is not available, write in the correct color next to the number. File the folders using the terminal digit system.

5/10/2010

ADMISSIONS	DOB	MR
Edgewater, Joan T.	6/12/1969	05-45-23
Jordan, Gina G.	7/9/1976	07-13-89
Ramirez, Maria M.	2/20/1985	06-45-63
Ramirez, Baby Girl	5/10/2009	06-45-64
Chen, Nancy O.	10/27/1979	05-75-94
Richards, Roger D.	8/19/1943	06-20-55
Bowers, Jonathan Q.	12/24/1930	06-07-71

DISCHARGES		MR
Jones, Samuel T.		4-56-24
Adams, George J.		06-12-12

5/11/2010

ADMISSIONS	DOB	MR
Soroczak, Angela P.	3/13/1953	06-45-65
Herrera, Sandra G.	10/30/1990	05-66-90

DISCHARGES		MR
Ramirez, Maria M.		06-45-63
Ramirez, Baby Girl		06-45-64

5/12/2010

ADMISSIONS	DOB	MR
Smith, Gordon M.	6/17/1971	06-45-66

DISCHARGES		MR
Edgewater, Joan T.		05-45-23
Richards, Roger D.		06-20-55
Chen, Nancy O.		05-75-94
Herrera, Sandra G.		05-66-90
Bowers, Jonathan Q.		06-07-71

8. What are thinned records and why are they important to the assembly process?

9. What are methods for searching for misfiles? Why is it important to know these methods?

10. What is the objective in record retrieval?

11. Discuss the differences of signing records in and out using a manual requisition system and a computer system.

Assembly of the Medical Record

Autopsy A postdeath examination of the body, including dissection of the internal organs, to determine the cause of death.

CBC Complete blood count.

CPT Current Procedural Terminology. Used to code procedures.

DRG Diagnosis Related Group. A group of diagnoses with similarities in treatment and resource consumption.

Differential diagnosis A tentative diagnosis, based on symptoms, made before any diagnostic tests are performed.

EKG Electrocardiogram.

ICD *International Classification of Diseases.* Used to code diagnoses and procedures.

Principal diagnosis The diagnosis that, after study, proves to be the reason for a patient's admission.

Respiratory and physical therapy Therapy to assist a patient with breathing and physical movement, respectively.

Secondary diagnosis An additional diagnosis which was treated or was present during the patient's hospitalization.

OBJECTIVES

When you have completed this chapter, you will be able to:

- Identify the different components of a medical record and their purposes.
- Discuss JCAHO and other regulatory agency requirements for medical record documentation.
- Discuss the purpose of reports found in obstetrical, psychiatric, and rehabilitation specialty records.

MEDICAL RECORD DOCUMENTS

When a patient is discharged from the hospital, the record is removed from its binder on the nursing station and delivered to the health information management department. Upon receipt, the record's documents are usually still in the order they were used on the nursing station. Because the needs of healthcare facilities differ, there is no one correct way to file the documents in a medical record. Each hospital develops its own chart order list that is used by the staff to file documents in the medical record. Having a specified order for the documents makes it easier for users of the record to find a specific document without searching through the entire record. In this chapter we will examine one way that the documents could be filed and look at the information that should be documented in each component. Figures 5.1 through 5.45 are copies of one patient's entire medical record. All identifying information has been deleted to maintain the confidentiality of the record.

FACE SHEET

The face sheet (Figure 5.1) is a document that contains demographic information about the patient, including name, address, age, sex, telephone number, attending physician, admitting diagnosis, and admission and discharge dates. The face sheet may also contain the **ICD** or **CPT** codes selected by the medical records coder, as well as the narrative descriptions of the final diagnoses and procedures. The purpose of the face sheet is to provide a quick reference about the hospitalization without having to delve further into the medical record. A copy of the face sheet is used by each physician who has treated the patient to collect data needed by his or her office for billing and record keeping. Providing copies of face sheets for physician offices is a common function of the HIM department.

SIGNATURE PROFILE

The signature profile (Figure 5.2) is a form on which each caregiver, except physicians, records his or her initials and full signature and title. Often the forms on which caregivers must document don't leave enough room for each person's full signature. Once the profile is completed, the caregiver may initial documentation instead. The profile also helps others reviewing the record to identify who the caregivers were. Not all hospitals use a signature profile.

DISCHARGE SUMMARY

The discharge summary (Figure 5.3) is the last document produced once a patient has been discharged from the hospital. Its purpose is to provide future users of the record with a brief synopsis of the patient's illness and treatment in the hospital. At a minimum it should contain the following information: admitting diagnosis, final diagnoses, reason for admission, pertinent clinical findings (for example, a test reveals that the patient has carcinoma of the breast), and significant laboratory findings. Significant laboratory findings mean only those laboratory values that are abnormal or that have a direct bearing on treatment of the patient. The entire result of any particular laboratory study need not be reiterated in the summary unless it is significant. The following sections describe additional information that will also be included in the summary.

Hospital Course

A chronological review of the patient's treatment starting with the first day and ending with the patient's discharge or death. It does not need to be as detailed as the actual progress notes the physicians write daily, and it should address only significant changes or improvements in the patient's treatment and condition.

Condition on Discharge

The condition of the patient at the time of discharge in relation to the condition of the patient at admission is noted. For example, if the patient was admitted with back pain, the condition on discharge should state whether the back pain was relieved, improved, or otherwise described.

Instructions to Patient and Family.   Instructions regarding diet, medications prescribed, and return visits to the physician's office are included in the summary. Physical limitations and their anticipated duration should also be specified if pertinent. Instructions may be documented on a separate form.

CODING SUMMARY

The coding summary (Figure 5.4) may be printed by the coder and placed in the record as a quick reference to the codes assigned and the resulting diagnosis related group, or **DRG.** Each DRG has a weight assigned to it that determines the reimbursement the hospital will receive for a Medicare patient with that DRG. Many other insurance companies use DRGs as statistical measures of the types of patients a hospital treats and as a guide to determining the reimbursement they will pay.

Determination of the DRG is made by entering the **principal** and **secondary diagnoses** and the major procedures into a computer, which then uses logic trees to arrive at the correct DRG.

PHYSICIAN ORDERS

Most hospitals have preprinted forms on which the physician lists his or her orders (Figures 5.5 to 5.9) for patient treatment. The admission order usually specifies the admitting diagnosis and such things as medications, type of diet, and treatment to be performed. If a consultation is required, the attending physician must order it in the physician order section. If the attending physician is going out of town or is transferring the care of the patient to another physician, he or she must write an order stating that he or she is no longer on the case and specifying the name of the physician who is taking over the care.

In order for the patient to be discharged, the attending physician must write a discharge order (Figure 5.5) specifying the day the patient is to be released. Orders may be handwritten by the physician or they may be taken over the telephone or verbally by a registered nurse (RN). A verbal or telephone order should be authenticated by the physician within the time frame specified by state law, usually 24 to 48 hours. Physician orders are filed in chronological order or reverse chronological order in the permanent record.

HISTORY AND PHYSICAL

The history and physical (H&P) is the first report to be completed when a patient is admitted to the hospital (Figure 5.10). Its purpose is to document the chief complaint of the patient, the **differential diagnosis,** and the initial proposed plan of treatment. The differential diagnosis is the tentative diagnosis made by the physician, based on the patient's symptoms, before any diagnostic tests are performed.

History

The history portion documents the following: *History of the Present Illness*—the length of time the patient has had the symptoms and what treatment, if any, has been tried on an outpatient basis. *History of Past Illness*—a review of major treatment received by the patient throughout his or her lifetime including any surgeries and significant illnesses. *Family History*—Medical information about the patient's family, including parents and siblings, which might be pertinent to treatment of the patient's illness. For example, if the patient has a family history of hypertension or diabetes mellitus, there may be strong indication for looking for those diseases in the patient. *Social History*—Aspects of the patient's lifestyle that might affect the diagnosis or treatment. It should include frequency of alcohol or tobacco use, religious or cultural beliefs, sleep habits, work, and stresses. *Review of Systems*—The physician asks the patient to relate any symptoms involving the six major body systems: (1) head, eyes, ears, nose, and throat; (2) chest/lungs; (3) gastrointestinal; (4) genitourinary; (5) musculoskeletal; and (6) neurologic. For example, in reviewing the gastrointestinal system, the physician may ask the patient if he or she has had any rectal bleeding, change in bowel habits, indigestion, and the like. In reviewing the genitourinary system, questions would be asked about urinary problems.

Physical

In the physical portion of the H&P, the physician documents the actual physical examination of the patient. The report starts with the head and goes through the body systematically as follows: (1) head, eyes, ears, nose, throat; (2) neck; (3) chest; (4) lungs; (5) heart; (6) abdomen; (7) genital/rectal; (8) skin; (9) extremities; and (10) neurologic.

The H&P ends with the differential diagnoses based on the patient's symptoms, plan of treatment, and prognosis.

CONSULTATION REPORTS

Often the patient's family physician, whose specialty may be family practice or internal medicine, admits the patient. When the nature of the illness requires the opinion of a specialist to assist with treatment, the attending physician will write an order for a consultation and will usually specify the name of the physician to be called. For example, if a patient is admitted after a fall with pain in the pelvic area and the x-ray reveals a fractured hip, the attending physician is likely to call in an orthopedic surgeon for consultation. The orthopedic surgeon would examine the patient and the patient's record and then dictate a report of the consultation.

Consultation reports document that the physician reviewed the patient's medical record for past medical history and other pertinent information, spoke to the patient about the illness, and examined the patient. The consultation report documents the consultant's findings, diagnosis, and recommendations for treatment. A very ill patient may have a number of different consultation reports in his or her medical record.

Surgical Consultation

If the patient must have surgery, the consultation report should specify that the physician discussed the surgery and any alternatives to surgery with the patient, including the risks involved in having the surgery and the benefits expected. It should also state that the surgeon feels the patient has given an informed consent to the surgery.

PROGRESS NOTES

Some hospitals use progress note forms that are used exclusively by the physician. Others use integrated progress notes in which all caregivers enter their progress notes in chronological order (Figures 5.11 to 5.18). It is important that each caregiver identify him- or herself by name and title to clarify to other caregivers and users of the record who has made the entry.

Frequency of Notes

Physician progress notes are usually handwritten. They are the day-to-day documentation of the patient's progress and treatment. The JCAHO requires that they be written as often as necessary to thoroughly document the patient's care. Usually this means that the physician will write at least one note per day in an acute care setting. If the patient is extremely ill, the physician may write more than one note daily.

Types of Notes

Progress notes may be filed in chronological order, starting with the patient's admission and ending with the discharge note, or left in reverse chronological order as they are on the nursing unit. The first note is usually made by the admitting physician and may parallel the dictated history and physical, in that it lists the patient's chief complaint, current symptoms, and the doctor's impression of the diagnosis and treatment being considered. Consultants usually write a brief note before dictating their consultation report. Surgeons are require to write a brief note (Figure 5.13) describing the surgery performed, immediately following the surgery.

CRITICAL CARE/SECOND VISIT NOTES

When a patient is treated in the intensive care unit, it may be necessary for a physician to visit the patient and perform a procedure or treatment more than once in a day. In order to provide accurate documentation for the record and for his or her billing purposes, some physicians dictate or write a critical care note or second visit note, which briefly documents why the physician saw the patient again and what treatment was rendered.

LABORATORY TEST RESULTS

During or prior to hospitalization, most patients will have some lab work performed. Most hospitals have computerized laboratory systems that print out results (Figure 5.19) for each patient. Results are printed daily, weekly, and as a final cumulative report after discharge. Only the final reports need to be maintained in the permanent medical record.

Manual Laboratory Reports

Manual laboratory test results are filed in chronological order by the type of test. A common type of laboratory mount form contains five to six columns of adhesive. Each lab report is affixed in chronological order to a separate adhesive column. The reports overlap with only the results of each showing. This type of form saves space in the record and allows the doctor or nurse to see changes in results quickly. For example, all urinalysis test results should be filed together, with the oldest report first and all the others shingled on top of it. Incorrect shingling of lab reports sometimes causes difficulties in photocopying and microfilming because not all report results can be read. Different types of laboratory reports should not be filed together on the same page. If the patient has one **CBC** report and one urinalysis report, the two should be filed on separate lab mount forms.

CANCER STAGING FORM

After a patient has been diagnosed with cancer, the cancer is staged by the surgeon or the oncologist, using the cancer staging form (Figure 5.20). Staging means that the cancer is assessed for size, lymph node involvement, pathology, presence of distant metastasis, and histopathology type and grade. Determining the stage of the cancer assists the physician in deciding upon treatment options. It also provides a way to compare cancer statistically.

PATHOLOGY REPORTS

Whenever a specimen is taken during surgery, it must be sent to the pathology department for analysis. The pathologist dictates the findings, and the transcribed report (Figure 5.21) is then placed in the medical record. The pathology report begins with a detailed description of the specimen, including color, texture, size, and other aspects of appearance. The body of the report contains the pathologist's findings, both gross and microscopic, and may include photographs of the cell type. The report ends with the pathologist's diagnosis based on the examination of the specimen. The pathologist may send specimens to other labs who provide specialized analysis (Figure 5.22).

RADIOLOGY REPORTS

Reports of x-rays, nuclear scans, CT scans, ultrasound, and other tests (Figure 5.23) are recorded in formats specific for radiology tests. Each type of test should be filed together. In a large hospital, these tests may be produced by individual departments. In a smaller hospital, the radiology department will usually be responsible for all of them.

CARDIOLOGY REPORTS

EKG results (Figure 5.24) are usually typed or computer printed on the actual EKG tracing and then filed in the record. Other types of reports, such as echocardiograms, have their own formats in which the results are recorded.

PROCEDURE/OPERATIVE REPORTS

The physician performing a procedure must prepare a report (Figure 5.25) documenting the preoperative diagnosis, the postoperative diagnosis, and the operation performed. The report describes the surgeon's findings upon opening up the patient.

This is followed by a detailed report of the procedure beginning with the first incision and ending with the closure. The report documents the type of sutures used and specifies the disposition of any specimens taken or tissue removed during the surgery. The operative report also states the names of the surgeon and the assistant surgeons.

ANESTHESIA DOCUMENTATION

Preanesthesia Note

During the surgical procedure, the anesthesiologist documents (Figure 5.28) the patient's vital signs, the type and dosage of the anesthetic, and the results of anesthesia. In addition to documenting during the procedure, the anesthesiologist is also required to document in a preanesthesia note (Figure 5.26) that he or she has examined and talked to the patient regarding the type of anesthesia to be used and has based that decision on the patient's past experience with anesthesia. The note should also document the patient's current physical condition and that the patient understands the risks associated with administering the anesthetic and consents to receiving anesthesia.

Postanesthesia Note

Within 24 hours following the surgery, the anesthesiologist must also write a postanesthesia note (Figure 5.27) in which he or she documents the results of an examination of the patient, including any complications or lack of complications from the anesthetic. This note must be dated and timed. Both the preanesthesia and postanesthesia notes are required by the Joint Commission on the Accreditation of Healthcare Organizations (JCAHO).

OPERATING ROOM CLINICAL RECORD

The operating room (OR) clinical record (Figure 5.29) is a form used by the OR nurses to document the preoperative diagnosis, the postoperative diagnosis, the planned procedure, and the procedure or procedures actually performed. It lists all equipment used during the operation, whether a sponge and instrument count was performed, and, if so, if they were correct. The form lists the names of all nurses involved in the surgery, the date, the time anesthesia was started, the operation start and end times, and the time anesthesia was ended. Some hospitals have computer systems in which to record this information.

POSTANESTHESIA CARE UNIT RECORD

The postanesthesia care unit (PACU) record form (Figure 5.30) contains documentation by the nurses in the recovery room of the patient's recovery from surgery. They document the patient's vital signs, fluids and medications given, and the patient's progress until he or she is ready to return to the regular nursing unit. The PACU record also documents the anesthesiologist's order for the patient's return to the nursing unit, or the use of preestablished discharge criteria by the nurse, and the time the patient was transferred.

$\mathscr{P}$REOPERATIVE PREPARATION RECORD

The preoperative preparation record (Figure 5.31) is a checklist of items that must be completed by nursing prior to the patient going to surgery. These include ensuring that the H&P is completed and recording vital signs.

$\mathscr{F}$ILING RELATED SURGICAL DOCUMENTS

There are two different ways to file the documents from consents to pathology reports, which we have described in the previous sections. The first involves filing the reports separately by type in date order. For example, all consents would be filed with the oldest first and the newest last.

Other hospitals file all the reports together for a particular procedure. For example, if a patient had an operation on September 9 and an operation on September 12, then the consent, the anesthesia record, the OR clinical record, the operative report, and the pathology report for the September 9 surgery would be filed together, followed by the reports pertaining to the second surgery.

$\mathscr{N}$URSING DOCUMENTATION

The JCAHO requires that caregiver documentation be multidisciplinary so that all of the needs of the patient are assessed and addressed. Even so, the majority of documentation falls to the nurses caring for the patient. The number and types of forms used for nursing documentation vary across the country.

Medication Administration Record

The medication administration record (Figures 5.32 to 5.34) documents each medication that is given to the patient. It includes documentation of the method of administration (e.g., intravenous [IV], intramuscular [IM], or subcutaneous [SC]); the site of the administration (e.g., left deltoid [LD] or right gluteus medius [RGM]); the dosage and frequency of administration ordered (e.g., 4 mg qid); and documentation of the actual time and date the medication was given as well as the initials of the nurse giving it. The form also requires the full signature of each nurse administering medication to the patient.

Nursing Database/Discharge Plan

The nursing database/discharge plan (Figure 5.35) is completed upon admission of the patient and is designed to record information about the patient that will assist the caregivers in providing specialized care for the patient. The nurse interviews the patient and records the patient's understanding of reason for hospitalization, allergies, vital signs, medical history, the patient's current medications, and the presence of an advance directive and/or organ donor card. Also recorded are the patient's personal history, social history, family history, cultural and religious preferences, primary language, and barriers to learning.

Discharge planning is begun by recording any type of assistance the patient receives at home; whether the patient can perform activities of daily living independently or needs help; whether the patient requires glasses, crutches, and the like; any anticipated need for assistance after discharge; and where the patient will be discharged to.

By recording this information at admission, no time is lost, for example, because an interpreter was not available for a patient who does not speak English. Or, discharge is not delayed because arrangements were not made for a hospital bed to be set up in the patient's home.

Graphic Patient Daily Care Sheet

The graphic daily care sheet (Figure 5.36) is used to record the patient's vital signs, intake and output, weight, activities, and appetite on a daily basis. Each sheet documents several days' information. The graphic format allows the caregivers visually to identify changes in the patient's status immediately.

Assessment Flow Sheet

The assessment flow sheet (Figure 5.37) allows the nurse to graph the daily assessments of each body system, and orders carried out, in a manner that easily identifies changes in the patient's status. In this form, the asterisk (*) indicates that there is a significant finding upon an order being carried out and the caregiver should see the integrated progress notes for more information. The arrow (→) indicates that the status is unchanged from the previous assessment. A check mark (✓) indicates that an order was carried out with no significant finding.

Admission Physical/Risk for Falls Assessment

The admission physical/risk for falls assessment (Figure 5.38) is a form used to record the patient's physical status at admission, by body system. A pain assessment is also recorded. The patient is also assessed by any conditions that might make the patient a greater risk for falling. Such conditions might include the patient's age and mental status. By assessing the patient upon admission, preventative measures can be taken to prevent falls.

Nursing Care Plans

Nursing care plans are required by the JCAHO as a mechanism to ensure that nursing care is focused toward the needs of each patient. The plan (Figure 5.39) identifies the focus of care (e.g., postoperative care), the expected outcomes (e.g., no evidence of wound inflammation/infection), and the plan for achieving the expected outcome (e.g., surgical dress/incision assessment).

Each different nursing unit will have a different care plan for the patient, including the postanesthesia recovery unit (Figure 5.30).

Teaching Record

The JCAHO requires documentation of patient teaching, including what was taught and to whom, and how the teacher knows that the patient has learned the material. Many hospitals have developed a form (Figure 5.40) to ensure that the required information is documented.

Nursing Discharge Status Note/Instruction Sheet

The nursing discharge status note/instruction sheet (Figure 5.41) serves two purposes. The first is to document the date and time of discharge, the patient's condition at discharge, and to where the patient was discharged. Second, it meets the JCAHO's requirement that discharge instructions to the patient be documented. Instructions include activity limitations, diet, signs and symptoms to watch for, medications, and follow-up appointments. Both the patient and the nurse giving the instructions sign the form.

*O*THER ANCILLARY REPORTS

Nutrition Services

The hospital dietician may use forms for documenting the number of calories that a patient has consumed over a specified time frame and for indicating diet counseling or assessment.

Respiratory Therapy and Physical Therapy

Therapists have specific forms (Figure 5.42) on which to document the date and frequency of the **respiratory and physical therapy** treatment given and the results of the treatment, along with any comments regarding the patient's status.

*C*ONSENTS

Whenever a patient undergoes any kind of invasive procedure, such as an appendectomy or chemotherapy, he or she must sign a consent (Figure 5.43) for that treatment. The documentation requirements for consent differ from state to state, but normally the consent will contain the attending physician's name, the surgeon's name, the name of the procedure in words understandable to a lay person not familiar with medical terminology, the date and time the consent is signed, the signature of the patient, and the signature and date of the witness. The consent may also specify the role of hospital personnel and the anesthesiologist in the performance of the procedure.

*C*ONDITIONS OF ADMISSION

The Conditions of Admission form (Figure 5.44) is signed by the patient at admission/registration. It allows the hospital to treat the patient and to perform minor diagnostic procedures, such as taking blood. The form is also an agreement that the patient will accept financial responsibility for the hospital bill. It must be signed by the patient or his or her guardian and is usually witnessed by a hospital employee.

*E*MERGENCY DEPARTMENT RECORD

The emergency department (ED) record (Figure 5.45) is the record of treatment received by a patient in the ED. The record usually contains demographic data about the patient, and it should specify how the patient arrived, that is, private car, ambulance, paramedics, police, or other means. Nursing personnel document the patient's chief complaint, vital signs, and any treatments, including medications, given in the ED. The ED physician documents the results the results of the physical examination, tests ordered, and an impression of the patient's problem. Many ED physicians dictate their reports.

Discharge from the ED

The ED record must state the condition of the patient on discharge from the ED in terms related to the patient's condition on admission. The record must also state the disposition of the patient—whether he or she went home, was transferred to another acute care facility, expired, or was admitted to the hospital. If the ED physician decides to admit the patient, the ED record becomes part of the inpatient record.

Patient Instructions

Most ED records contain a separate document on which the physician records instructions for follow-up treatment. For example, if the patient has had a head injury, there will be instructions on the symptoms of concussion and what to do if any of them occur. The follow-up instructions may also tell the patient to return to the ED to be checked again in a specified number of days or to see his or her own private physician.

Paramedic Report

If the patient is brought in by the paramedics, the paramedic report becomes a part of the ED record. It will include the condition of the patient upon the paramedics' arrival, what resuscitative methods or other treatment they used, and any drugs that they gave the patient.

RECORD OF DEATH

The record of death form (Figure 5.46) is completed when a patient expires. It usually contains the patient's name, address, age, the date and time of death, the name of the physician who pronounced the patient dead, and the cause of death as determined by the attending physician. It may also contain a section that is signed when the body is turned over to the mortuary for funeral arrangements.

AUTOPSY REPORT

When a patient expires, the family is asked if they will agree to a postmortem examination (**autopsy**). If they do agree, or if the death is a coroner's case in which an autopsy is required by law, a report of the examination is generated. The autopsy report states the pathologist's determination as to the cause of death and gives a detailed description of all body systems as they are examined, including the weight and condition of all major organs.

TRANSFER RECORD

When a patient is admitted to a small community hospital, he or she may require treatment not available at that hospital and must be transferred to an acute care facility with more extensive services. For example, a patient admitted with an acute myocardial infarction may need to be transferred to another facility that performs cardiac catheterizations to determine the extent of the coronary artery blockage. A patient who no longer needs acute care may be transferred to a nursing home. Or, a resident at a nursing home may need to be transferred to the hospital for acute care. In any of these cases, a transfer form (Figure 5.47) must be completed to document the circumstances of the transfer. The form will document the name and address of the hospital transferring the patient; the patient's name, age, and diagnosis; the name and address of the facility receiving the patient; and the reason for the transfer. A copy of the completed transfer form is sent along with the patient, to be placed in the receiving hospital's medical records.

OB/NEWBORN RECORD

Prenatal Records

During pregnancy the expectant mother visits her obstetrician periodically for examinations. Records of these visits are called prenatal records. When the patient is near her delivery date, the physician's office sends the original or a copy of the prenatal records to the hospital where they will be included in the medical record. Prenatal records are very specific about the woman's past pregnancy history, including any miscarriages and previous deliveries. Because prenatal records include a history and physical, the physician may not be required to dictate a history and physical when the patient is admitted in labor. However, the physical examination portion should be updated at the time the patient actually arrives to be delivered. The prenatal records are usually filed in the same area of the record where the dictated history and physical would be found. A dictated H&P is required prior to a Cesarean section.

Perinatal Testing

When an expectant mother goes into premature labor or has any other complications of the pregnancy, the obstetrician may order a nonstress test to determine if there is fetal distress. These tests are performed on an outpatient basis, and the results are included as part of the medical record when the woman actually comes into the hospital to deliver.

Preprinted Pre- and Postpartum Orders

Many obstetricians have specific orders that they use on all patients. In this case the hospital will usually preprint these orders so that all the physician has to do is sign the form and make any changes that might be specific to a particular patient. Preprinted orders should be filed in the record with the other physician orders.

Labor and Delivery Records

The labor record is the documentation of the patient's condition during labor, including any medications given, any monitors applied, any fetal distress noted, and the like. The delivery record (Figure 5.48) specifies the date and time of delivery; the sex of the child; the type of delivery, including Cesarean section or vaginal delivery; position of the fetus (e.g., breech); type of laceration, if any, and repair made; the time the placenta was expelled; and other information pertinent to the delivery. The delivery record also includes the Apgar scores at 1 and 5 minutes. In the Apgar rating system, the baby's color, heart rate, respiratory effort, muscle tone, and reflex irritability are rated on a scale from 1 to 10 by the physician at 1 minute and 5 minutes after birth.

Newborn Physical Exam

Once the newborn has been transferred from the delivery room to the nursery, the pediatrician will examine the baby to ensure that there are no abnormalities or problems. This exam is usually documented on a form (Figure 5.49) designed so the physician checks off whether each body part is normal or abnormal. If the pediatrician discovers an abnormal finding, he or she must then further document the abnormality.

Footprint and Armband Certification

A footprint, like a fingerprint, is unique for each person. In many facilities, newborns are footprinted as a means of identifying the child. The armband is placed on the newborn immediately after birth, and the number on the armband corresponds with the number on the mother's armband. At the time the mother takes the baby home, she must sign a certification that she has examined the baby's armband and that the number matches that on her armband. This certification, along with the footprints, is filed in the medical record.

Postpartum Teaching Record

Some obstetrical units have a checkoff form in which the nurses document that the mother has been taught and has successfully demonstrated how to do such things as bathing the baby, breastfeeding, and changing a diaper.

R EHABILITATION RECORDS

Often patients who have had strokes or other types of brain or spinal injuries require rehabilitation before they can function normally. Hospitals that specialize in rehabilitation treatment have some forms in their records that may be different from acute care records.

Therapy Records

Therapy records document the type of therapy given, the frequency, and the patient's response to the therapy. These are filed in chronological order in the record.

Team Conference Notes

Team conference notes are the documentation of weekly conferences that all members of the treatment team attend. The team members could include the attending physician, counselors, different types of therapists, and social services personnel. The purpose of the conference is for all members of the team to discuss the patient's diagnosis and prognosis, plan the treatment to be given, and discuss the results of that treatment. These forms should also be filed in chronological order.

P SYCHIATRIC RECORDS

Patients with psychiatric diagnoses, including substance abuse, are usually treated with a multidisciplinary approach. A treatment team, consisting of the attending physician, psychologist, nurses, counselors, and social workers, meets on a periodic basis to discuss the patient's diagnosis, prognosis, treatment, and response to treatment. The treatment plan is the form on which the information discussed at the meetings is recorded.

Group Therapy Notes

A portion of the treatment involves group therapy in which the patient interacts with other patients and/or family members. The counselors conducting the group therapy session make progress notes regarding what was discussed and how the patient reacted or contributed to the discussion. The group therapy notes may be on separate forms, which should be filed in chronological order, or they may be part of the integrated progress notes.

Pass Consent

Because a patient undergoing treatment may be in the hospital quite some time, he or she may be allowed to go home for one to two days. In order to do this, the patient or his or her guardian must sign a consent to allow a "pass." The consent states that the hospital has no liability while the patient is away from the hospital.

Psychological Assessment/Testing

Other reports that may be seen are the records of psychological assessment and/or psychological testing, which are conducted by a psychologist. These reports are dictated and will normally be found in the same section as consultation reports.

PERMANENT DIVIDERS

In an effort to utilize medical record staff and time more efficiently, some hospitals have decided to use permanent dividers in the medical records. Each component of the medical record, many of which we have discussed, such as physician orders, history and physical, medication records, laboratory reports, and progress notes, is given a separate divider. The dividers are placed in the inpatient binder, and the individual records are placed behind the appropriate divider during the hospitalization.

Upon discharge, the entire record, including the dividers, is removed from the binder, and the record is sent to the health information management department. Because the dividers identify each part of the record, further assembly is no longer necessary. The dividers can be customized according to the individual hospital's need, and different sets of dividers are usually made for different types of records. For example, acute medical/surgical records would have specific dividers, as would obstetrical records and newborn records.

Some hospitals recycle the dividers back to the nursing units to save money.

_____ _____ Medical Center

```
                                MEDICAL CENTER
                           INPATIENT ADMISSION
                       --------------------------
                                                    : MRU:      - -
                                                    : CASE:
   924 E JUNEAU #705          MRST: SINGLE    SEX: F : ADMT: 10/24/
                             DOB: 05/10/1937 ( 60 Y) :      19:11
   PHN:                       RLGN: EPISCOPALIAN      --------------------
   SSN:                       RACE: 4 - 2             CAMPUS:        -E
                                                     BED: N46101
                                                     UNIT: 4N
                                                     SVC: SUR
                                                     ACCOM: S
COMPLAINT: RIGHT BREAST CANCER                    ADM TYP: ELECTIVE

PROCED: 10/24/97   INJURY: NONE         DT: NONE

PHYS: ADMIT: 1575         , WILLIAM L   (UPIN:        )
      ATTND: 1575         , WILLIAM L   (UPIN:        )
      REFER:
      PERSN:
      ROLE1:
  ** PAT EMPLOYMENT (FOR OOY)  **        ** CONTACT ** (RELATION:    COUSIN
OCC: NONE
EMP: NONE                                      534 N 115 ST

                                          PHN:
                                          ALT: UNKNOWN
                                         ** CONTACT 2 ** (RELATION: BROTHER

                                              PHN:
                                              ALT: UNKNOWN

   ** GUARANTOR **  (RELATION:    SELF        )


   PHN:
   ALT: UNKNOWN

PRI. INS: M01-MEDICARE
   INS NO:                        SSN:
   PATIENT HAS: PART A/B BENEFITS  EFFECTIVE DT: 10/01/88
   LAST HOSP: 11/11 1111



SEC. INS: B05-BLUE CROSS OUT-OF-ST        SUBSCRIBER (RELATION:    SELF      )
                                                              SSN:
                                          EMPLOYER:
                                  EFF FR:   / /
   POL:                               TO:  / /
   GRP NO:                        GRP NAME:
   TREATMENT AUTH:
COMMENT:

                                       PRINTED BY: DLP      PRINTED:
                                                            10/24/
```

FIGURE 5.1 Face sheet.

Medical Center

SIGNATURE PROFILE

Please sign your full signature, title and initials when
documenting on this patient's record.

DS 1022 MR - -
M02,805 SCE
W. 1575
C5-10-37 60 F

Date	Initials	Signature and Title	Date	Initials	Signature and Title
			10-22-97	AL	
			10/24/97	9	KM
			10-24-97	AB	Kn
			10-24-97	CJ	APCA
			10-25	DL	RN
			10-25	CJ	APCA
			10-25-97	RL	APCA
			10/25/97	W,H	APCA
			10/25	BS	
			10/25	NS	
			10-25-97	Ae	APCA.

05100870*

SIGNATURE PROFILE

FIGURE 5.2 Signature profile.

<u>**Medical Center**</u>

```
        MED. REC. NO.:  00-
            PT. NAME:                     ,
                 DOB:  05/10/1937
                   D:  10/26/
                       William L.          , MD
        HOSP. NO.:
```

DATE OF ADMISSION: 10/24/
DATE OF DISCHARGE: 10/26/

DIAGNOSIS(ES): Right breast carcinoma.

SURGERY PERFORMED: Right lumpectomy with axillary node dissection on the right side.

PAST MEDICAL HISTORY AND REASON FOR ADMISSION: Patient is a 60-year-old white female who was admitted for invasive carcinoma of the right breast. This was found as a palpable upper outer quadrant mammographic mass composed of closely adjacent 10 mm and 5 mm nodules on 10/07/ . It was diagnosed with an ultrasound-guided core biopsy on 10/09/ . EKG, UA, CBC, chemistries, chest x-ray and bone scan were all normal. She wished breast conservation.

Past medical history is significant for Charcot-Marie-Tooth disease.

Past surgical history is significant for tendon transplants for bilateral foot drop, left breast biopsy and bilateral mastoidectomies.

She is on no medication at home. She discontinued hormone replacement therapy approximately one week ago after ten years of treatment.

She has PENICILLIN and SULFA allergies.

Physical exam showed a normally developed white female with normal heart and lung sounds. She had a soft and nontender abdomen. She had no supraclavicular or left axillary adenopathy. She had an upper outer quadrant radial scar on the left breast and a 2.0 cm vague mass on the upper outer quadrant of the right breast. She had mobile clinically suspicious node in the right axilla.

ADMISSION DIAGNOSIS(ES): Invasive ductal carcinoma of the right breast, T1, N1, M0, stage 2.

The plan was for right segmental mastectomy and a right axillary lymph node dissection on the day of admission. Patient underwent this procedure on 10/24/ without incident. She tolerated the procedure well without any problems. Her postoperative course was unremarkable. She remained afebrile and was tolerating a regular diet before discharge. Her JP drain output was between 100 and 200 cc a day, therefore, the drain will be left in place, to be taken out at a later

Page 1 of 2   **DISCHARGE SUMMARY**

                                                              ORIGINAL

FIGURE 5.3 Discharge summary.

Medical Center

MED. REC. NO.: 00- - -
PT. NAME:
DOB: 05/10/1937
D: 10/26/
William L. , MD
HOSP. NO.:

date as an outpatient. Her incisions were clean, dry and intact, and she is ambulating without difficulty. Patient will be seen in Dr. clinic in approximately three days, at which time her wounds will be checked and her dressings changed.

William L. , MD

Dictated By: Jeanne , MD
JC/nmv DT: 10/29/ DD: 10/26/ D#: 185001

cc: Jeanne , MD
William L. , MD

Page 2 of 2 **DISCHARGE SUMMARY**

ORIGINAL

FIGURE 5.3 Continued.

```
                              MEDICAL CENTER
                            BILLING OFFICE FORM
                          FOR MEDICARE A PATIENTS

PATIENT NAME . . . . .          '
ADMISSION DATE . . . . 10/24/          DISCHARGE DATE . . . . 10/26/
MEDICAL RECORD # . . .                 DATE OF BIRTH . . . . 05/10/37
AGE . . . . . . . . . 60               SEX . . . . . . . . . F
BILLING NUMBER . . . . 00000           SOCIAL SECURITY #. . .      -   -
SOP . . . . . . . . . M  MEDICARE A


DX1   174.4  MAL NEO BREAST UP-OUTER      PR1  #85.21 LOCAL EXCIS BREAST LES
                                          PR2  *40.3  REGIONAL LYMPH NODE EXC







ATTENDING PHYS . . . . 1575          , WILLIAM L.
CONSULTING PHYS. . . .
OTHER PHYS . . . . . .

10/24/   1575               , WILLIAM L.  10/24/   1575              , WILLIAM L.


I    OSITION. . . . . . 01 - HOME (ROUTINE)
LOS = 002                  GEOM. MEAN LOS =  1.4            LOS TRIM PT = 00
MDC = 09                   DRG WEIGHT = 0.6092
DRG = 260  SUBTOTAL MASTECTOMY FOR MALIGNANCY W/O CC
TOTAL CHARGES = $      0   ANCILLARY CHARGES = $       0
REIMBURSEMENT = $4018

                         *** LOS OUTLIER ***

STATUS . . . . . . . . . . . I
CODER: GD
DATE:  10/31/
```

FIGURE 5.4 Coding summary.

PHYSICIAN'S ORDER SHEET
MEDICAL CENTER

WHEN NO NUMBER SHOWS IN THE CIRCLE, CHANGE FORMS

<u>USE BALL POINT PEN ONLY</u>

PRESS HARD YOU ARE MAKING TWO COPIES

```
IP 1024        MR  -  -
               M01.B05 SCE
05/10/37   V L
           60      F        1575
```

ALLERGIES:

PCN, Sulfa

PHYSICIAN'S ORDERS (EXCLUDING MEDICATION ORDERS)	MEDICATION ORDERS ONLY ANOTHER BRAND OF GENERICALLY EQUIVALENT PRODUCT, IDENTICAL IN DOSAGE FORM AND CONTENT OF ACTIVE INGREDIENT MAY BE ADMINISTERED WHEN INDICATED.

DATE 10/26/

Discharge when cleared
per Dr

JP drainage teaching
— empty + record perm

F/u Dr   Tues/Wed
              call for appt
leave brn on, daily
    dressing changes

                        MD

              09^10 10/26/

MEDICATION ORDERS

DATE   TIME

Rx Percocet

R.N. _____   M.D. _____

DATE   TIME

R.N. _____   M.D. _____

DATE   TIME

10-26-

1. no daily dressing changes
2. Discharge today —
3. Give Rx for pain —

              1300
                 10/26/9?

R.N. _____   M.D. _____

05200590

FIGURE 5.5 Physician orders.

PHYSICIAN'S ORDER SHEET
MEDICAL CENTER

IP 1024   HR

MO1.B05 SCE

05/10/37   W L   60   F   1575

WHEN NO NUMBER SHOWS IN THE CIRCLE, CHANGE FORMS

ALLERGIES:

PCN, Sulfa

USE BALL POINT PEN ONLY

PRESS HARD YOU ARE MAKING TWO COPIES

| PHYSICIAN'S ORDERS (EXCLUDING MEDICATION ORDERS) | MEDICATION ORDERS ONLY | ANOTHER BRAND OF GENERICALLY EQUIVALENT PRODUCT, IDENTICAL IN DOSAGE FORM AND CONTENT OF ACTIVE INGREDIENT MAY BE ADMINISTERED WHEN INDICATED. |

DATE 10/25

① D/c O₂

② D/c IV

③ D/c Teds

④ Ambulate q shift

⑤ Teach pt how to record
Drain output + take
daily temperatures

⑥ D/c LVF.

M 7502

elem 1500, 10/25

10-25

no more antibiotics

pulled 10/10/01

05200590

FIGURE 5.6 Physician orders.

_____ Medical Center

POST ANESTHESIA CARE UNIT ORDERS
— Place (✓) next to orders which apply
— Fill in blanks as necessary
— Only orders CHECKED and FILLED IN will be carried out

NURSING CARE

☑ Blood pressure, pulse, respirations on admission and q15''
☑ Temperature on admission and discharge
☑ EKG monitoring upon admission and through discharge
☐ Arterial, CVP, and PA monitoring when applicable
☑ Pulse oximetry upon admission through discharge

> ☐ Wrist   R   L }
> ☐ Vest/Jacket   }   Restraints for _____ behavior for duration of PACU stay.

RESPIRATORY CARE

☑ Humidified O_2 by mask at 10Lpm.
☐ 40% aerosol at 10Lpm by mask/T-piece/ETT.
☐ O_2 per nasal cannula at_____Lpm.
☐ May extubate when the following parameters are met:
   A. Awake
   B. Lifts and holds heads off bed for 5 seconds, cough reflex present, squeezes hand on command.
   C. Adequate V_T, V_M, F.V.C.
☐ ET tube to ventilator V_T_____cc FIO_2_____ Rate_____
☐ Extubation and weaning orders for patients on ventilators must be obtained from anesthsiologist.

> ☐ If patient unable to maintain O_2 Sat of_____, order nasal canula at _____ L/min till _____.
> Check O_2 SAT on room air. If $\geq$ 90% D/C the oxygen. If < 90% call surgeon.

MEDICATIONS

☐ I.V. Rate per surgeon's orders.
☐ If no I.V. orders, keep 1 line open with 1L of last infused solution.
☐ Acute hypotension, I.V. rate increased, notify M.D.
☐ In the absence of a physician, the following emergency orders will be followed:
   1. When PVC's occur more than 6/min., on the preceding T-wave, are coupled or multifocal in nature, give lidocaine 50mg I.V. STAT. May repeat x1 in 5''.
   2. If arrythmia above persists, start an infusion of 2GM lidocaine in 500 D5/W, not to exceed 2 mg/min.
   3. If PVC's persist after 20-30'', give lidocaine 50 mg I.V.
   4. When cardiac rate is less than 50 and patient is symptomatic, give atropine 0.5mg I.V. May repeat x 1.
   5. When any of the above occur, notify surgeon and anesthesiologist

DIAGNOSTIC STUDIES

☐ ABG's
   ☐ STAT on admission with H+H, K, and sodium
   ☐ 20'' after ventilator change, start on T-piece, or extubation
   ☐ PRN in PACU
☐ H+ H _____'' after transfusion.
☐ Glucose upon admission.

DISCHARGE

☑ Return to floor after____/____'' and/or VS stable q15'' x 2 Aldrete 7+
☐ Check with anesthesiologist for specific discharge order.

ADDITIONAL ORDERS: _Demerol 50mgm "Im" if needed_
for pain _____

X4693 (Rev. 8/95) - 61 fc   Signature _____   Date _____

NOTE: These orders in effect only through PACU stay.

FIGURE 5.7 Physician orders.

PHYSICIAN'S ORDER SHEET

MEDICAL CENTER

WHEN NO NUMBER SHOWS IN THE CIRCLE, CHANGE FORMS

USE BALL POINT PEN ONLY

PRESS HARD YOU ARE MAKING TWO COPIES

DS 1024. MR - -
MC2,805 SCE
W L 1575
05/10/37 63 F

ALLERGIES:
None

PHYSICIAN'S ORDERS (EXCLUDING MEDICATION ORDERS)

DATE 10-24-
NPO
Apply long TED stockings pre op
Void on call to the OR
Send to nuclear medicine for 10:15 isotope injection.
Send to Breast Health Center for 11:00 localization.
Consent for right segmental mastectomy and right axillary lymph node dissection.
Right modified radical mastectomy only if necessary. Also node mapping procedure

William L. MD

10/24/ 6pm
To 4N Dr
vitals q 1° x4 then q shift
up tonight only c assistance
Clears when awake, Advance As tolerated
IS to bedside, use 10x q° WA
If no void by 10³⁰ pm, straight cath
Strip JP q shift + prn & empty & Record
Do not change dressings.
HUC 10/[illegible]
MA

MEDICATION ORDERS ONLY ANOTHER BRAND OF GENERICALLY EQUIVALENT PRODUCT, IDENTICAL IN DOSAGE FORM AND CONTENT OF ACTIVE INGREDIENT MAY BE ADMINISTERED WHEN INDICATED.

DATE TIME

1

R.N. M.D.

DATE 10/24 TIME 1845
O_2 per nasal cannual
at 3 L/min till Am.
Check O_2 SAT on room air.
[illegible]
If ≤ 90% call [illegible]
P.O. of [illegible]
R.N. M.D.

DATE TIME
IV: D5 45 NS @ 100 cc/°
Erythromycin 500 mg IV q 8° (due c 2200) X 3 doses
MSO4 2-4 mg IV q1° prn
Compazine 10mg IV q 6° prn SLOWLY
Percocet i-ii PO q 4° prn pain
10/24 0100
R.N. M.D.

05200590

FIGURE 5.8 Physician orders.

PHYSICIAN'S ORDER SHEET
Medical Center

D   1022.   MR   -   -
              M02,305   SCE
              , W.   1575
ALLERGIES: 1 - 37   60   F

USE BALL POINT PEN ONLY
PRESS HARD YOU ARE MAKING TWO COPIES

PHYSICIAN'S ORDERS *(EXCLUDING MEDICATION ORDERS)*		MEDICATION ORDERS ONLY		
DATE:	TIME:	DATE	TIME	

Admit to A.S.C.

CONSENT for: *Rt. Seg. Mast + Axillary Node Dissection*

☒ NPO

☒ CBC with Diff ✗   *4 R*

☐ POTASSIUM (If on diuretic)

☐ GLUCOSE (If diabetic)

☒ CHEM ⑥ 7, ⑫ ✗   *4 R*

☐ HIV

☐ PT, PTT, BLEEDING TIME

☐ RPR

☒ U/A - with MICRO ✗   *4 R*

☐ URINE PREGNANCY TEST (on admit)

☒ EKG (required on age 40 and over)   *4 R*

☒ CHEST XRAY (if clinically necessary) ✓   *R*

☐ TYPE AND SCREEN/CROSS # of units_____

☒ HISTORY AND PHYSICAL *from Dr.*   *gc*

☐ FLEETS ENEMA

☐ SEQUENTIAL STOCKINGS

☐ TED STOCKINGS KNEE/THIGH HIGH

☐ CIRCUMFERENTIAL SURGEX PREP:

☐ ____ Inches above and inches below_____

☐ Knee, ankle, elbow, hip, shoulder

☐ Crutchwalking Instructions.

☐ Other:_____

Verbal

Pre printed Orders per:

Dr._

X4637

PHYSICIANS ORDER - Admit to A.S.C.

R.N.		M.D.

FIGURE 5.9 Physician orders.

Breast   Initial   Evaluation   (typed)

Date of Examination___10/21/_____

Name_____ Age_____60___ Race___W___ Sex___F___

Chief   Complaint:_____Invasive carcinoma of the right breast_____

Present   Illness: Patient stated that she saw Dr.   for an annual breast examination
on 10/7/ . She was unaware of any problems with her breasts but a mammogram showed a poorly
defined lobulated mass measuring 1.4x1.2 cm in diameter in the upper outer quadrant of the right
breast. A 1.5 cm firm mass was palpable at the 10:30 o'clock position in the right breast. A
hand-held ultrasound showed two hypoechoic masses in the upper outer quadrant of the right breast
measuring 1 cm and .5 cm. She was recalled and on 10/9/ . an ultrasound-guided core biopsies
were performed of the two adjacent mass in the upper outer quadrant. Both showed invasive
carcinoma. Patient said she is now aware of the lump in her right breast. She does not perform
bse regularly but she has had previous mammograms and ultrasound examination and understood that
the mammogram a year ago was normal. She has been told she has cystic disease on the basis of
previous examinations but is asymptomatic with respect to her breast. She had been taking hormone replacement therapy for the last ten years but stopped it one week ago after the present
problem became known. She has experienced no recent symptoms of bone or joint pain, headache,
dizzy spells or chest pain.

Past   History

   Illnesses___Charcot-Marie tooth disease_____

   Operations_____Tendon transplants for drop foot in 1986 and 1987; bilateral mastoidectomies
      left breast biopsy in 1984, benign_____

   Allergies_____Penicillin and sulfa_____

   Medications_____None_____

   Hormones/OCs_____Estrace one mg qd; Provera 2.5 mg qd for the last ten years until one week
   Hx of Irradiation Treatment_____None_____
                            ago

Review   of   Systems

   Gravida_0_____ Para_____0_____ LMP____1984_____ Menarche ___11_____

   Age first pregnancy _____ Age first Childbirth _____

   Other_____Review of systems generally unremarkable._____

   _____

   Tobacco,Alcohol,Drugs____She quit smoking ten years ago after a ten pack year history; no
                            alcohol intake

Family   History

   Breast   Cancer_____Maternal aunt had breast cancer ten years ago_____

   Other   Cancer_____Maternal grandmother had liver cancer; maternal aunt had leukemia;
                       brother had prostate cancer; an uncle had liver cancer

   X-Rays & Slides ____Mammograms Breast Diagnostic Clinic 10/7/ with magnification compression
   views and an ultrasound examination of the left breast 10/7/   showing two masses in the upper
   outer quadrant of the left breast, one 10 mm and the other 5 mm in diameter, very close to each
   other. She also brought slides from   Memorial Hospital S-9647-97_____

FIGURE 5.10 History and physical.

Physical Examination

General   Description_____Normally developed, white female_____

Height (in.)__66.5"___ Wt (lbs)__167 lbs___ BP 156/94 rt arm**Pulse**___60_____
                                                    154/100 left arm

Head   and   Neck____Not remarkable_____

Lungs_____Clear to P&A_____

Heart___Regualr rhythm, no murmurs_____

Abdomen____Soft and nontender_____

Extremities___No pretibial edema; thighs were not examined_____

Lymph   nodes:___No supraclavicular adenopathy ,and no left axillary adenopathy; vague
mass felt high in the right axilla
   her/Rectal/Pelvic____._____

Breasts Medium and symmetric with no nipple inversion. A radial scar is present in the
upper outer quadrant of the left breast. The left breast is soft and nontender, no nipple discharge could be expressed. In the low axillary part of the right breast a healing puncture wound
was evident. In the upper outer quadrant of the right breast a vague deep perhaps 2 cm mass
could be felt but the finding was subtle. I felt no masses elsewhere and could express no nipple
discharge. The left axilla was clinically negative. In the right axilla there appeared to be
an enlarged lymph node in the mid to high axilla which was clinically suspicious.

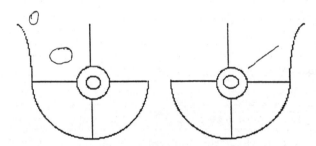

Impression/Diagnosis__Invasive carcinoma of the right breast; two foci closely adjacent_
   in the upper outer quadrant, clinically T1N1M0

Disposition/Plan   I reviewed the mammograms and ultrasound examination and will review
the slides with our pathologist for confirmation. I discussed the diagnosis with the patient
and recommended either breast conserving therapy or modified radical mastectomy. I explained
these two procedures and she wished to be treated with breast conservation, indicated the
hazards of lymphedema of the right arm or susceptibility to infection. She was given information
on the pros and cons of both approaches and information about hospitalization. Preoperative and
imaging studies were scheduled. She was anxious to get started with treatment because of wishing
to leave for Florida in the next month. A tentative date for surgery was scheduled. She will
be tentatively scheduled for a right lumpectomy, right axillary lymph node dissection. It may be
necessary to localize the right breast tumor preoperatively and I indicated that node mapping
may also be part of the procedure. She was in agreement.
                         Signature_Cu_____ _____

FIGURE 5.10 Continued.

ATTENDING ADMISSION NOTE
MEDICAL CENTER

DATE	NOTES
10-24-	This 60 year old white female is admitted for
	CC/ Invasive carcinoma of the right breast
	CC/ This was found as a palpable UOQ mammographic mass
	composed of closely adjacent 10 mm and 5 mm nodules on 10-7- and
	was diagnosed with US guided core biopsy on 10-9- . Her EKG, UA,
	CBC, SMA-6&12, CXR and bone scan are normal. She wishes breast
	conservation.
	PMH/ Illnesses=Charcot-Marie Tooth disease. Ops= Tendon
	transplants for foot drop, lt br bx, bilat mastoidectomies. Meds=None;
	quit HRT one week ago after 10 years of Rx. NO ALLERGIES.
	ROS/NR Mat aunt had breast CA
	PE/ Normally developed white female. Wt=167 Lbs, BP= 156/94
	H&N= NR Heart and lung sounds normal. Abdomen soft and nontender.
	No supraclavicular or left axillary adenopathy. UOQ radial scar on lt
	breast. 2.0 cm vague mass in UOQ of right breast. Mobile clin suspicious
	node in rt axilla. No pretibial edema; thighs not examined.
	DX/ Invasive ductal carcinoma of the right breast. T1N1M0 Stage II
	PLAN/ Right segmental mastectomy and right axillary lymph node
	dissection on day of admission.
	William I . MD

05100660   ATTENDING ADMISSION NOTE

FIGURE 5.11 Progress notes.

_____ Medical Center

PATIENT PROGRESS NOTE

```
C9  1022      MR   -   -
             M02,A05  SCE
             W.  1575
C5-10-37   60 F
```

Date/Time	Focus	D = Data A = Action R = Response
10/22/ 1415	labs	D- Chem6+12 WNL, CBC-WNL, UA-I abnormals A-labs faxed to Dr — R
10/25/	Chest 4/S Completed 0910 L Ashrun RDMS	
10-25- 1149 A	localization completed — W	

PATIENT PROGRESS NOTE

FIGURE 5.12 Progress notes.

MEDICAL CENTER

05/10/37   62   F   1575

PROGRESS NOTES - SPECIAL

DATE	POST OPERATIVE NOTES	NOTES
10/24/97	SURGEON: Dr.	
	ASSISTANTS: Dr. JMS	
	ANESTHETIC: General	
	PRE-OPERATIVE DIAGNOSIS: Infiltrating ductal CA of (R) breast	
	POST OPERATIVE DIAGNOSIS: Same	
	OPERATION PERFORMED: Lumpectomy and axillary node dissection level I & II	
	DRAINS: (R) Axillary JP drain 15 F BLOOD LOSS: 200 cc	

BLOOD USE: Ø

Please indicate # used:
Whole   Packed
Blood _____   Cells _____   Platelets _____   FFP _____   Cryo _____   Alb _____

Indication for Blood/Blood Product Use:

PATIENT CONDITION: Stable to recovery

JMS

_____ M.D.

05200340

PROGRESS NOTES · SPECIAL

FIGURE 5.13 Progress notes.

_____ Medical Center

10 2\.

OS 1024   MR - -
                M02,B05 SCE
              . W L   1575
OS/10/37 60   F

PATIENT PROGRESS NOTE

Date/Time	Focus	D = Data A = Action R = Response
10/24/ 1005	Transfer	A: To Nuclear Medicine in stable condition ambulatory. R2
10/24/ 1645	BHC	To nuclear med p̄ local per Dr. _____ OR at 1330. Pt. tolerated injection of methylene blue. Pt. stable. ⊖ RN
10/24 1915	Post-op	D: Pt. transferred from recovery via bed by 2 RN's; IV infusing, pt. stable at this time.
	Neuro	D: Sleepy, but easily arousable. ———
	CV	D: Fair tachycardic. See graphics. ———
	Resp	D: ↓breath sounds in bases bil. on 3L O₂ per NC. ———
	Pain	D: c/o incisional pain, rated 10/10. A: Given morphine IV 4mg.
	GU	D: DTV post-op.
	GI	D: Tolerating sips of H₂O ⊕ bowel sounds.
	MS	D: Assist of ↑ for bed mobility. ↓ROM RUE 2° surgery. ——— RN
10-24-		2215 hr Off ward, Awake + VS OK Dressing intact, sips of H₂O + has not voided LW

PATIENT PROGRESS NOTE

FIGURE 5.14 Progress notes.

PATIENT PROGRESS NOTE

Date/Time	Focus	D = Data A = Action R = Response
10/24	GU	D: Voided blue colored urine c̄ difficulty.
2215	GI	D: ⊕ bowel sounds. Ø c/o N/V. Tolerating cl. liq. + crackers.
	MS	D: Amb. c̄ 1 assist. ↓ ROM Ⓡ UE. weakness in arms + legs 2° hx of Charcot–Marie Tooth disease; has bilat. foot drop.
10/25	09:15	General Surgery
		S: Pod #1 s/p Ⓡ Lumpectomy c̄ Axillary LN Resection. Doing well. Ø c/o minor incisional pain / discomfort. Ambulating in hall c̄ assistance. Tolerating general diet. Denies tingling / numbness, loss of strength in Ⓡ UE.
		O: T_M = 98.4 T_c = 98.0 HR = 91–111 BP = 120–150/70–85 RR = 20 I/O = 1993 / 1230 + 80 JP drain over 16 hr General: awake, alert. Ø apparent discomfort / distress. RUE: wound C/D/I. Steri-strips in place. Ø sign of infxn. Good strength. ROM to = clavicle.
		A/P: Pt is Pod #1 s/p Lumpectomy c̄ Axillary LN dissection. Doing well. Hemodynamically stable. Afebrile. ① ✓ Pain control — cont d/ percocets ② d/c Ted stockings ③ d/c IV ④ Encourage ambulation prn
		Af VSS wound looks good good ROM Ⓡ arm Tolerating PO intake Ambulating Doing well d/c PVI

FIGURE 5.15 Progress notes.

Medical Center _____

PATIENT PROGRESS NOTE

I P	MR
	M01,B05 SCE
05/10/37 60 F	**1575**

Date/Time	Focus	D = Data A = Action R = Response
		RESPIRATORY CARE DEPT.
		Date _10/25/_
		Doctor _____ :
		To meet criteria for reimbursement, oximetry or blood gases are required on patients receiving oxygen therapy within 24 hours of initiation of therapy and every 96 hours thereafter. To help us comply, please order either oximetry or an ABG.

RESPIRATORY CARE DEPT.
DOCTOR

OXIMETRY DONE: DATE: _10/25/_
___ EAR
_✓_ PULSE   TIME: _0930_
ROOM AIR SATURATION: _95_ ___%
O₂ @ ____ LPM SATURATION: ____ %
COMMENT: _87HR_
Tech: _Q,_

O₂ _DC'ed_

10-25-   1st _Pod_

Afebrile
IV removed + dressing D'ed
Incisions OK
cut

PATIENT PROGRESS NOTE

FIGURE 5.16 Progress notes.

PATIENT PROGRESS NOTE

Date/Time	Focus	D = Data A = Action R = Response
10/25/ 13[00]	RESP	D: O_2 SAT = 95% ON ROOM AIR.
		A: O_2 @ 3L DC'ED PER MD ORDER.
	GI	D: ADVANCED TO GEN. DIET s̄ NAUSEA, ⊕ FLATUS BUT
		⊖ POST-OP BM. RW
10/25/ 2130	Resp	D ↓ BS bilateral bases
10/26/ 06[30]	JMS PN	General Surgery
		Pt. s̄ complaints pain is controlled by medication
		Tm 99^6 Tc 98^3 VSS
		I/O ~~2344~~ 3774/2747 JP 97cc ∅ stool
		heart: RRR
		lungs CTA Ⓑ
		abd soft, NT, ND, ⊕ BS
		RUE good ROM, incisions c/d/i drain intact
		A/P POD#2 s/p Lumpectomy & Axillary node dissection
		① Pt. has not had a BM will consider a stool softener prn
		② Pain controlled by medication
		MS
10/26/ 0830	JP	D: JP HOME DRAINAGE TEACHING IN PROGRESS.
		A: REFAMILIARIZED PATIENT IN JP DRAINAGE INSTRUCTIONS;
		FYWB ON JP HOME DRAINAGE GIVEN.
		R: MS. HAD NO QUESTIONS; APPEARS NO
		PROBLEMS c̄ SELF-DRAINAGE; RECORDING AT THIS
		TIME. WILL OBSERVE PATIENT IN 2 HRS. DOING
		PROCEDURE ON OWN. RW

05200000* pg. 2-38 **PATIENT PROGRESS NOTE**

FIGURE 5.17 Progress notes.

Medical Center

IP MR
M01.B05 SCE
1575
05/10/37 60 F

PATIENT PROGRESS NOTE

Date/Time	Focus	D = Data A = Action R = Response
10/26/		Surgery VSS AF doing well pain controlled. tolerating po / Ambulating Feels ready for d/c today JP teaching [illegible]
10/26/ 1030	JP	R: PERFORMED JP DRAINAGE & RECORDING 100% ON OWN s̄ PROMPTING OR CUES. ANTICIPATE Ø PROBLEMS c̄ JP CARES @ HOME. PATIENT VERBALIZES SECURITY c̄ DOING JP CARE ON OWN @ HOME. RN
10-26-		2nd Pod — Dressing changed + incisions OK Discharged c̄ Ax drains. Rx given for percocet To be seen in office in 2 days [illegible]

▯ X 5 3 4 2 ▯

05200000*

PATIENT PROGRESS NOTE

FIGURE 5.18 Progress notes.

```
10/23/                    HEALTH CARE LABORATORIES          OUTPATIENT FINAL CUM SUMMARY
22:55              LABORATORY MEDICINE -                              PAGE 1

------------------------------------------------------------------------------------------


NAME:
MR #:                      DOB: 05/10/37            DR:
LOC:   SCE                 AGE: 60Y
ROOM:                      SEX: F
ACCT:


       ---------------------------- HEMATOLOGY AUTOMATED CBC ----------------------------------
TEST:        WBC        RBC        HGB        HCT      PLTC      MCV      MCH      MCHC     RDWSD     MPV
UNITS:       K/UL       M/UL       G/DL        %       K/UL      FL       PG       G/DL      FL       FL
LO-HI:     4.0-11.0   3.85-5.28  12.0-14.7   34-44   140-400   78-97    26-34    32-36    39-47   8.9-11.0

10/22/
#   0753      6.3        4.80       14.4        42      213        87      30       35        43      11.0

                          ------------- HEMATOLOGY AUTOMATED CBC -------------
TEST:        NEUT       LYMPH      MONO        EOS      BASO
UNITS:        %          %          %          %        %
LO-HI:       45-80      15-45      0-11        0-6      0-2

10/22/
#   0753      53         35         10          2        0

       --------------------------------------- CHEMISTRY-1 -------------------------------------
TEST:      GLUCOSE      NA         K          CL       HCO3      BUN    CREATININE
UNITS:      MG/DL     MMOL/L    MMOL/L     MMOL/L    MMOL/L    MG/DL     MG/DL
LO-HI:      65-115    135-145    3.5-5.0    98-107    23-32    10-20     0.6-1.1

10/22/
#   0753       99        142        4.6        105       30       13        0.9

       --------------------------------------- CHEMISTRY-2 -------------------------------------
TEST:        AST        ALT        LD       ALK PHOS  BILI TOTAL  URIC ACID  CHOLESTEROL
UNITS:       U/L        U/L        U/L        U/L      MG/DL       MG/DL       MG/DL
LO-HI:      15-46      11-66     313-618     38-126    0.2-1.3     2.5-7.5      <200

10/22/
#   0753       21         35        504         62        0.6         6.0        186

              ------------------------------- CHEMISTRY-2 -------------------------------
TEST:     PHOSPHORUS   CALCIUM   T. PROTEIN  ALBUMIN
UNITS:      MG/DL      MG/DL       G/DL       G/DL
LO-HI:     2.5-4.5    8.8-10.2    6.0-8.2    3.5-5.0

10/22/
#   0753      3.6         9.7        6.9        4.1




                              CONTINUED                              PAGE 1
                                                       OUTPATIENT FINAL CUM SUMMARY




05400500
```

FIGURE 5.19 Laboratory report.

```
   10/23/                 HEALTH CARE LABORATORIES          OUTPATIENT FINAL CUM SUMMARY
   22:55              LABORATORY MEDICINE -                            PAGE 2

---------------------------------------------------------------------------------------


   NAME:
   MR #:                      DOB: 05/10/37           DR:
   LOC:    SCE                AGE: 60Y
   ROOM:                      SEX: F
   ACCT:


         ~~~~~~~~~~~~~~~~~~~~~~~~~~~~~~~~~~~ URINALYSIS SCREEN ~~~~~~~~~~~~~~~~~~~~~~~~~~~~~~~~~
   TEST:        COLOR   APPEARANCE      GLU   BILI   KET   SPEC GRAV    BLD     PH     PROT
   UNITS:                               MG/DL        MG/DL                             MG/DL
   LO-HI:       YEL                     <100  NEG    <5    1.005-1.030  NEG   5.0-7.0   <15
        _____
   10/22/
   #   0735   STRAW   CLEAR            NEG   NEG    NEG    1.010      SMALL    7.0     NEG
                                    _____ URINALYSIS SCREEN _____
   TEST:        URO     NIT   LEUK
   UNITS:       EU/DL
   LO-HI:      0 1.0   NEG    NEG
        _____
   10/22/
   #   0735    0.2    NEG    NEG
         ~~~~~~~~~~~~~~~~~~~~~~~~~~~~~~~~~~~ URINE MICROSCOPIC EXAM ~~~~~~~~~~~~~~~~~~~~~~~~~~~~~~
   TEST:        RBC'S          WBC'S         EPI'S       BACTERIA     HYAL
                                                                      CASTS
   UNITS:       /HPF           /HPF          /HPF        /HPF         /LPF
   LO-HI:       0-2            0-5           1-3                      0-2
        _____
   10/22/
   #   0735   3 TO 5        0 TO 2        3 TO 5     NONE SEEN   NONE SEEN
```

```
                            END OF REPORT                         PAGE 2
                                                       OUTPATIENT FINAL CUM SUMMARY
```

05400500

FIGURE 5.19 Continued.

BREAST

Data Form for Cancer Staging   **Oncology Record**

Patient Identification

Name_____   Anatomic site of cancer_____

Address_____   Histologic type_____

Hospital or Clinic Number_____   Grade (G)_____

Age _____ Sex _____ Race_____   Date of classification_____

Clin	Path		
			DEFINITIONS
			Primary Tumor (T)
[ ]	[ ]	TX	Primary tumor cannot be assessed
[ ]	[ ]	T0	No evidence of primary tumor
[ ]	[ ]	Tis	Carcinoma *in situ*: Intraductal carcinoma, lobular carcinoma *in situ*, or Paget's disease of the nipple with no tumor
[ ]	[ ]	T1	Tumor 2 cm or less in greatest dimension
[ ]	[ ]	pT1mic	Microinvasion 0.1 cm or less in greatest dimension
[ ]	[ ]	T1a	Tumor more than 0.1 cm but not more than 0.5 cm in greatest dimension
[ ]	[ ]	T1b	More than 0.5 cm but not more than 1 cm in greatest dimension
[✓]	[✓]	T1c	More than 1 cm but not more than 2 cm in greatest dimension
[ ]	[ ]	T2	Tumor more than 2 cm but not more than 5 cm in greatest dimension
[ ]	[ ]	T3	Tumor more than 5 cm in greatest dimension
[ ]	[ ]	T4	Tumor of any size with direct extension to (a) chest wall or (b) skin, only as described below
[ ]	[ ]	T4a	Extension to chest wall
[ ]	[ ]	T4b	Edema (including peau d'orange) or ulceration of the skin of breast or satellite skin nodules confined to same breast
[ ]	[ ]	T4c	Both (T4a and T4b)
[ ]	[ ]	T4d	Inflammatory carcinoma

Paget's disease associated with a tumor is classified according to the size of the tumor.

Regional Lymph Nodes (N)

Clin	Path		
[ ]	[ ]	NX	Regional lymph nodes cannot be assessed (e.g., previously removed)
[✓]	[✓]	N0	No regional lymph node metastasis
[ ]	[ ]	N1	Spread to movable ipsilateral axillary lymph node(s)
[ ]	[ ]	N2	Spread to ipsilateral axillary lymph node(s) fixed to one another or to other structures
[ ]	[ ]	N3	Spread to ipsilateral internal mammary lymph node(s)

Pathologic Classification (pN)

Clin	Path		
	[ ]	pNX	Regional lymph nodes cannot be assessed (e.g., previously removed, or not removed for pathologic study)
	[✓]	pN0	No regional lymph node metastasis
	[ ]	pN1	Metastasis to movable ipsilateral axillary lymph node(s)
	[ ]	pN1a	Only micrometastasis (none larger than 0.2 cm)
	[ ]	pN1b	Metastasis to lymph nodes, any larger than 0.2 cm
	[ ]	pN1bi	Metastasis in 1 to 3 lymph nodes, any more than 0.2 cm and all less than 2 cm in greatest dimension
	[ ]	pN1bii	Metastasis 4 or more lymph nodes, any more than 0.2 cm and all less than 2 cm in greatest dimension
	[ ]	pN1biii	Extension of tumor beyond the capsule of a lymph node metastasis less then 2 cm in greatest dimension
	[ ]	pN1biv	Metastasis to a lymph node 2 cm or more in greatest dimension
	[ ]	pN2	Metastasis to ipsilateral axillary lymph nodes that are fixed to one another or to other structures
	[ ]	pN3	Metastasis to ipsilateral internal mammary lymph node(s)

Distant Metastasis (M)

Clin	Path		
[ ]	[ ]	MX	Distant metastasis cannot be assessed
[✓]	[ ]	M0	No distant metastasis
[ ]	[ ]	M1	Distant metastasis (includes metastasis to ipsilateral supraclavicular lymph node(s))

(continued on next page)

CANCER STAGING
BREAST

Reference: American Joint Committee on Cancer - 1997

FIGURE 5.20 Cancer staging form.

BREAST *(continued)*

Clin	Path		Stage Grouping			
[ ]	[ ]	0	Tis	N0	M0	
[ ]	[ ]	I	T1*	N0	M0	
[✓]	[✓]	IIA	T0	N1	M0	
			T1*	N1**	M0	
			T2	N0	M0	
[ ]	[ ]	IIB	T2	N1	M0	
			T3	N0	M0	
[ ]	[ ]	IIIA	T0	N2	M0	
			T1*	N2	M0	
			T2	N2	M0	
			T3	N1	M0	
			T3	N2	M0	
[ ]	[ ]	IIIB	T4	Any N	M0	
			Any T	N3	M1	
[ ]	[ ]	IV	Any T	Any N	M1	

* T1 includes pTmic.
**The prognosis of patients with N1a is similar to that of patients with pN0

Staged by_____ **Managing M.D.**

_____ **Pathology, M.D.**

_____ **Registrar**

Date___11-22_____

Illustrations

REGIONAL LYMPH NODES

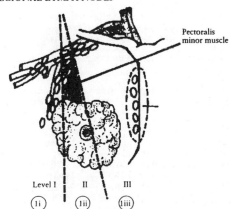

Pectoralis
minor muscle

Level I   II   III
(1i)   (1ii)   (1iii)

Histopathologic Grade (G)

[ ]	GX	Grade cannot be assessed
[ ]	G1	Well differentiated
[ ]	G2	Moderately differentiated
[ ]	G3	Poorly differentiated
[ ]	G4	Undifferentiated

Histopathologic Type

The histologic types are the following:

Carcinoma, NOS (not otherwise specified)
Ductal
   Intraductal (in situ)
   Invasive with predominant intraductal component
   Invasive, NOS (not otherwise specified)
   Comedo
   Inflammatory
   Medullary with lymphocytic infiltrate
   Mucinous (colloid)
   Papillary
   Scirrhous
   Tubular
   Other
Lobular
   In situ
   Invasive with predominant *in situ* component
   Invasive
Nipple
   Paget's disease, NOS (not otherwise specified)
   Paget's disease with intraductal carcinoma
   Paget's disease with invasive ductal carcinoma
Other
   Undifferentiated carcinoma

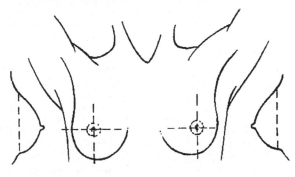

Indicate on diagram primary tumor and regional nodes involved.

FIGURE 5.20 Continued.

LABORATORIES
Medical Center

CASE NUMBER:

                                                    DR:

NAME:
ACCT #:
MR #:   MS

```
-----------------------------------------------------------------------
                            SURGICAL REPORT
-----------------------------------------------------------------------
```

LOC:
AGE/SEX: 60Y F   DATE COLL: 10/24/
DOB: 05/10/1937   DATE RECD: 10/25/

ORDERING DR:

COPY TO: X-RAY

SPECIMEN: RIGHT BREAST BIOPSY
                 NEW DEEP MARGIN
                 SENTINEL LYMPH NODE RIGHT AXILLA
                 POSSIBLE SENTINEL LYMPH NODE RIGHT AXILLA
                 POSSIBLE SENTINEL LYMPH NODE RIGHT AXILLA
                 AXILLARY NODES LEVELS 1 AND 2

CLINICAL DIAGNOSIS: Right breast carcinoma

```
-----------------------------------------------------------------------
```

GROSS EXAMINATION:
A - The specimen consists of a right breast measuring 7.5 x 5.0 x 1.5 cm
in greatest dimension. The specimen is inked as follows: the entire
deep margin is inked in blue, the medial margin is inked in green, the
superficial margin is inked in black and the lateral margin is inked in
red. The specimen is serially sectioned and a 1.5 cm nodule noted near
the deep resection margin within < 1.0 mm of the blue ink is found near
the medial inferior aspect of the tissue submitted. A portion is
submitted for frozen section labeled "FS1". The remaining lesion is
submitted from medial to lateral in cassettes labeled #1 through #7.
The second lesion measuring 1.0 cm in greatest dimension, (that first
nodule is 1.5 cm in greatest dimension), the second one is 1.0 cm in
greatest dimension is located within < 1.0 mm of the deep margin on the
inferior lateral aspect. It is submitted as "FS2". The remaining
portions of tissue from the area of the lesion are submitted in
cassettes #8 through #12.
KWS:kk
B - The specimen received in formalin labeled "new deep margin-black ink
on surgical margin" is a portion of muscle 3.5 x 2.5 x 1.5 cm with a cat
gut suture coming from the non-blackened side. The specimen is
sectioned in multiple transverse sections and submitted in its entirety.
C - The specimen received in formalin labeled "sentinel lymph node right
axilla" is a firm irregular reniform portion of yellow-tan nodal tissue
1.5 x 1.0 x 0.8 cm. It is surrounded by soft yellow lobules of fat.
The node is multiply sectioned and embedded in its entirety.
D - The specimen received in formalin labeled "possible sentinel lymph
node right axilla" is an irregular portion of yellow lobular adipose
tissue which is 5.5 x 1.5 x 0.5 cm. Within it is a 0.5 cm in diameter
lymph node. The entire specimen is embedded.

DEPARTMENT OF LABORATORY MEDICINE

FIGURE 5.21 Pathology report.

PAGE 2

E - The specimen received in formalin labeled "possible sentinel lymph node right axilla #3" is an irregular, roughly ovoid lymph node surrounded by fibroadipose tissue. The purple firm nodal tissue is 1.0 cm in greatest dimension. The entire specimen is embedded.
F - The specimen received in formalin labeled "axillary nodes level I and II chromic on apex" is an irregular but roughly triangular portion of fibrofatty tissue 15.0 cm in height x 9.0 cm at the base and 3.0 cm in greatest thickness. The specimen is dissected for the presence of lymph nodes beginning at the apical portion and lymph nodes as they are found are placed sequentially in cassettes #1 through #6 with two bisected lymph nodes placed in cassette #4, a single lymph node cut into multiple sections in #5 and #6.
JEW:kk

OPERATING ROOM CONSULTATION:
AFS1 - Frozen Section Diagnosis: Infiltrating duct cell carcinoma.
      (PJH/KWS)
AFS2 - Frozen Section Diagnosis: Infiltrating duct cell carcinoma.(PJH)
      (PJH/KWS)

MICROSCOPIC DESCRIPTION:
A - Permanent sections confirm the frozen section diagnosis. The sections demonstrate two foci of moderately differentiated ductal carcinoma. Tubule formation is noted in approximately 20% of each focus. The neoplastic cells exhibit moderate nuclear pleomorphism with occasional distinct nucleoli. Tumor is not seen at the inked margins, but does approach within 1 mm of the deep margin. Definite lymphovascular invasion by tumor is not identified. A minor component of intraductal carcinoma is seen, predominantly of the solid and cribriform type with an intermediate nuclear grade. Mitotic figures are rare and average less than one per ten high power fields. The non-neoplastic breast exhibits proliferative fibrocystic change. Ductal epithelial proliferation is florid in a few ducts.
B - Sections of the specimen submitted as new deep margin show unremarkable skeletal muscle with no evidence of invasive carcinoma.
C - Sections of the specimen submitted as sentinel lymph nodes show no evidence of metastatic carcinoma.
D - Sections of the specimen submitted as possible sentinel lymph node show no evidence of metastatic carcinoma.
E - Sections submitted also as possible sentinel lymph node show no evidence of metastatic carcinoma.
F - Sections demonstrate 15 lymph nodes with no evidence of metastatic carcinoma. There is prominent sinus histiocytosis with fibrosis.

DIAGNOSIS:
A - RIGHT BREAST BIOPSY:
      1.   MULTIFOCAL INFILTRATING MODERATELY DIFFERENTIATED DUCTAL
           CARCINOMA (1.5 AND 1.0 CM IN GREATEST DIMENSION), MODIFIED
           BLOOM-RICHARDSON GRADE II/III.
      2.   SURGICAL MARGINS FREE OF TUMOR (DEEP MARGIN <1 MM).
      3.   MINOR COMPONENT OF DUCTAL CARCINOMA IN SITU, SOLID AND
           CRIBRIFORM TYPE, INTERMEDIATE GRADE.
      4.   NO DEFINITE EVIDENCE OF LYMPHOVASCULAR INVOLVEMENT BY TUMOR.
      5.   FOCALLY FLORID PROLIFERATIVE FIBROCYSTIC CHANGE.
      6.   BREAST PROGNOSTIC STUDIES SUBMITTED. AN ADDENDUM TO FOLLOW.
B - SKELETAL MUSCLE, SPECIMEN SUBMITTED AS NEW DEEP MARGIN, EXCISION:
    NO EVIDENCE OF INVASIVE CARCINOMA.
C - SENTINEL LYMPH NODE, RIGHT AXILLA, EXCISIONAL BIOPSY: NO EVIDENCE
    OF METASTATIC CARCINOMA.

DEPARTMENT OF LABORATORY MEDICINE

FIGURE 5.21 Continued.

```
D - POSSIBLE SENTINEL LYMPH NODE, RIGHT AXILLA, EXCISIONAL BIOPSY:  NO
    EVIDENCE OF METASTATIC CARCINOMA.
E - POSSIBLE SENTINEL LYMPH NODE, RIGHT AXILLA, EXCISIONAL BIOPSY:  NO
    EVIDENCE OF METASTATIC CARCINOMA.
F - LYMPH NODES, LEVELS 1 AND 2, RIGHT AXILLARY DISSECTION:  NO EVIDENCE
    OF METASTATIC CARCINOMA IN 15 IDENTIFIED LYMPH NODES (0/15).
(4)


                    ***** ADDENDUM *****

RESULTS OF RECEPTOR AND PROLIFERATIVE MARKER ANALYSES (FROM SEPARATE
FLOW CYTOMETRY REPORT DN97-335):

ESTROGEN:                   POSITIVE (MODERATE-STRONG)
PROGESTERONE:               POSITIVE (MODERATE-STRONG)
C-erbB-2 ONCOPROTEIN:       EQUIVOCAL
DNA INDEX/PLOIDY:           1.1/ANEUPLOID
S-PHASE FRACTION:           6.2%


            , M.D.
PATHOLOGIST


10/27/  :11/7/
CPT: 88307X2, 88305X4, 88331, 88332;ICD-9: 174.9
END OF REPORT
```

DEPARTMENT OF LABORATORY MEDICINE

FIGURE 5.21 Continued.

Laboratories
Medical Center/

CASE NUMBER:

                       DR:

NAME: COPY TO:

ACCT#:

MRU#:   MS   SOURCE: RIGHT BREAST

                                   (DNAP)

LOC: DATE RECD: 10/28/

DOB: 05/10/1937   AGE/SEX: 60Y F

BREAST CANCER PROFILE

MARKER	RESULT	FAVORABLE INDICATOR
Estrogen Receptor:	POSITIVE (MODERATE-STRONG)	Positive
Progesterone Receptor:	POSITIVE (MODERATE-STRONG)	Positive
C-erbB-2 Oncoprotein:	EQUIVOCAL	Negative

(Immunohistochemistry performed at   Memorial Hospital)

DNA CONTENT ANALYSIS

DNA Index/Ploidy	1.1/ANEUPLOID	Normal = Diploid
S-phase Fraction	6.2%	Normal = <8.0%

November 5,   (db)   , M. D.

CPT4 88182, W88342(x3) ICD-9 174.9

ModFit Cell Cycle Analysis

File: C:\TEMP\p04rv007.
Patient: DN97-335
Acc #: S97-4207-A6
Tissue: R BREAST,TUMOR

%DIPLOID: 55.16
   %Dip G0-G1: 97.22 at 205.52
   %Dip G2-M: 2.78 at 411.04
   %Dip S: G2/G1: 2.00
   %Dip CV: 5.99
%ANEUPLOID1: 44.84
   %An1 G0-G1: 31.11 at 230.20
   %An1 G2-M: 55.10 at 479.78
   %An1 S: 13.79 G2/G1: 2.08
   %An1 CV: 2.26 DI: 1.12

Total %S-Phase: 6.18
%Debris: 17.75 %Aggregates:
Total Events: 17140.89 RCS: 1.528

%Diploid B.A.D.: 8.82

%Aneuploid B.A.D.: 12.34

%Total B.A.D.: 8.97

■ SingleCut Deb
■ Dip G0-G1
■ Dip G2-M
☐ An1 G0-G1
☐ An1 G2-M
▨ An1 S

Cells (y-axis): 100, 200

DNA Content (x-axis): 120, 240, 360, 480, 600, 720, 840, 960

05300380

DEPARTMENT OF LABORATORY MEDICINE

FIGURE 5.22 Specialized pathology report.

Medical Center

MED. REC. NO.:
PT. NAME:
DOB: 05/10/1937
ROOM NO.:   SCE
ATTENDING PHYS.:   , MD
HOSP. NO.:

```
ORDERING PHYSICIAN:                    , MD

DATE OF EXAM:  10/24/

TYPE OF EXAM:  RIGHT BREAST LOCALIZATION

The examination was conducted by the attending physician, Dr.          .

An area of dense tissue in the right axillary area was localized with
needle.  Iodinated contrast material was also used.

        DT:  10/31/   DD:  10/30/   D#:  185521

cc:                   , MD
```

_____
                                          , MD

Radiology Consultation

ORIGINAL

FIGURE 5.23 Radiology report.

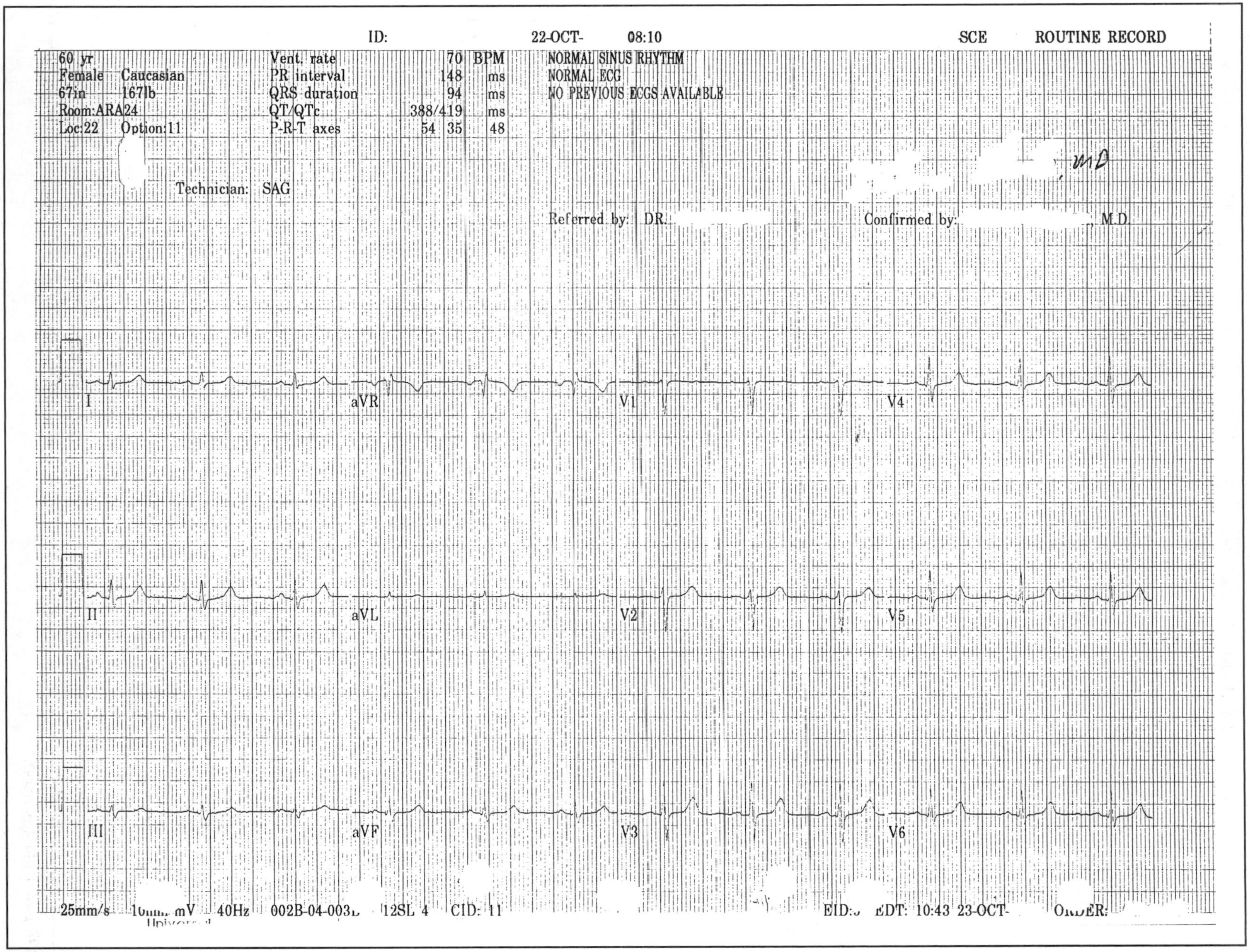

FIGURE 5.24 EKG

<u>**Medical Center**</u>

MED. REC. NO.:
PT. NAME:
DOB: 05/10/1937
ROOM NO.:   N46101
, MD

HOSP. NO.:

SURGEON: , MD

1ST ASST: , MD

2ND ASST: , MS

ANESTHESIA: General endotracheal

DATE OF PROCEDURE: 10/24/

PREOPERATIVE DIAGNOSIS(ES):
Invasive ductal carcinoma of the right breast.

POSTOPERATIVE DIAGNOSIS(ES):
Invasive ductal carcinoma of the right breast.

NAME OF PROCEDURE(S):
RIGHT SIDE MIDDLE MASTECTOMY AND RIGHT AXILLARY LYMPH NODE DISSECTION,
LEVELS I AND II, WITH NODE MAPPING AND SENTINEL NODE BIOPSY.

PRELIMINARY NOTE: This is a 60-year-old white female who was found on
mammogram to have a suspicious mass in the upper outer quadrant of the
right breast.   This was diagnosed with a core biopsy that was
ultrasound-guided on 10/09/ , and she chose to be treated with breast
conservation.   Preoperatively, 800 uCi of technetium sulfa colloid was
injected into the right breast for node mapping, and a localization
procedure was performed on the right breast because a mass was only
vaguely palpable, and more precision was needed.

OPERATIVE PROCEDURE(S):   The patient was given 500 mg of Erythromycin,
and the skin was prepared with Betadine soap, Betadine solution, and
draped sterilely, so that only the breast was exposed.   A curvilinear
incision was made in the upper outer quadrant of the right breast,
directly over the suspected site of the mass, and carried down through
the superficial subcutaneous tissue.   At this point, a mass could be
more clearly felt, and it was widely excised down to the pectoralis
major muscle.   The specimen was tagged to orient the pathologist using
black silk sutures.   The pathologist's report was two nodules of
invasive ductal carcinoma, and all margins were free of tumor.   The
tumor was within 1 mm of the deep margin, so at this point, the
pectoralis major muscle that was in the depths so that the biopsy cavity
was removed, as a new deep margin, the new surgical margin was stained
with blue day and the specimen was submitted for permanent sections.

Page 1 of 3   **OPERATIVE/PROCEDURE REPORT**

                                                    ORIGINAL

FIGURE 5.25 Operative report.

<u>**Medical Center**</u>

```
          MED. REC. NO.:
            PT. NAME:
                DOB:  05/10/1937
            ROOM NO.:  N46101
                                        , MD
            HOSP. NO.:
```

Hemostasis was electrocautery, and the incision was closed with 3-0 chromic catgut interrupted sutures to the subcutaneous tissues and running 4-0 Prolene subcuticular pull-out suture to the skin. Steri-Strips were applied. The overdrape was removed, and after a change of gowns, gloves and instruments, the breast was draped from the field to expose only the axilla. The curvilinear incision was made in the right axilla in the skin lines, and carried to the axillary fashion. A superior flap was developed up to the superior axillary fold, and an inferior tapering flap was dissected distally. Before the breast incision had been closed, 4 cc of Lymphazurin had been injected into the walls of the segmental mastectomy cavity, and at this point of the axillary dissection, blue dye-stained tissue in lymphatics was looked for. Some blue-stained breast tissue was identified, but no definite blue-stained lymphatics however. Using a gamma probe, it was possible to identify three radioactive lymph nodes which were removed as sentinel lymph nodes numbers 1, 2, and 3; and these were submitted separately. a scan of the remaining axilla revealed no residual radial activity. The gamma probe used was the C-scan. Next, the bleeding border of the latissimus dorsi muscle was exposed, and the lateral border of the pectoralis major muscle was exposed. It was noted that the resected portion of the pectoralis major muscle did appear in the lower end of the axillary wound. The pectoralis minor muscle was then exposed preserving the lateral pectoral nerve that ran over his lateral margin. Then the axillary vein was identified and cleaned along its lower margin, dividing its inferior tributaries between hemoclips. The vein was traced under the pectoralis minor muscle, and the axillary tissues deep to the pectoralis minor went up to its medial margin were dissected free from the chest wall and moved laterally. The intercostal brachial nerve was identified at this point and was traced out into the arm, preserving it along its length. As the dissection proceeded, the long thoracic nerve was identified and preserved, as was the thoracodorsal nerve and the thoracodorsal vessel. All the node-bearing tissues surrounding the structures were dissected en bloc and finally removed by dividing the remaining attachments to the lower skin flap. The wound was irrigated with warm saline. Then a 15-French round fluted Blake-type drain was placed in the axillary wound, and exited distally. It was attached to a Jackson-Pratt reservoir. The incision was then closed with 3-0 chromic catgut sutures to the subcutaneous tissues, and a running 4-0 Prolene subcuticular pull-out suture to the skin. Decompression was good. Steri-Strips were applied, and then fluff dressing was applied over the axillary incision and the breast incision using a surgi-bra to hold them in place. A sterile dressing was applied around the drain site. The sponge count was correct. The patient

Page 2 of 3   **OPERATIVE/PROCEDURE REPORT**

ORIGINAL

FIGURE 5.25 Continued.

Medical Center

MED. REC. NO.:
PT. NAME:
        DOB: 05/10/1937
ROOM NO.:   N46101
                                                    , MD
HOSP. NO.:

received no blood. She tolerated the operation well, and left the operating suite in satisfactory condition.

_____
                                                          , MD

        DT: 10/24/   DD: 10/24/   D#: 183243

CC: , MD
                                 , MD

Page 3 of 3   **OPERATIVE/PROCEDURE REPORT**

                                                              ORIGINAL

FIGURE 5.25 Continued.

Medical Center

D S   M R
            M02,805   SCE
              1575
C5-10-37   60 F

ANESTHESIA DEPARTMENT

PRE-ANESTHETIC EVALUATION

10-24 ℞ Mastectomy

PRIOR ANESTHETICS AND COMPLICATIONS
- [x] none *GA in past week tolerated*
- [ ] respiratory *No family hx of anesthetic complications*
- [ ] headache
- [ ] prolonged emergence
- [ ] nausea *PSHx: Mastoid surgery (childhood)*
- [ ] vomiting *Bilat lower extremity tendon transfer*
- [ ] fever *Tonsillectomy (1957)*
- [ ] other _____

CARDIOVASCULAR *Denies CAD, exercise intolerance*
- [x] none
- [ ] angina
- [ ] arrhythmias
- [ ] infarction
- [ ] other _____
- [ ] CAD
- [ ] hypertension
- [ ] CHF
- [ ] valvular disease

CNS / NEUROMUSCULAR ✗
- [ ] none
- [ ] seizures
- [ ] stroke
- [ ] arthritis
- [ ] other ✗ *CHARCOT - MARIE TOOTH SYNDROME (upper + lower extremity muscle weakness)*
- [ ] OBS
- [ ] myopathy
- [ ] spinal surgery / trauma
- [ ] neuropathy *No cardiac/respiratory muscle involvement*

(a form of muscular dystrophy)

RESPIRATORY
- [ ] none
- [ ] asthma
- [ ] bronchitis
- [ ] URI
- [ ] occupational
- [ ] emphysema
- [ ] ~~smoker~~ *NONSMOKER Quit 10 years ago*
- [ ] dyspnea
- [ ] cough
- [ ] COPD
- [ ] atelectasis
- [ ] other _____

AIRWAY EVALUATION
- [x] normal *MPTI I Good thyromental distance*
- [ ] other _____ *Neck flexion ≥ 15°*

CLASSIFICATION
- [ ] 1
- [x] 2
- [ ] 3
- [ ] 4
- [ ] 5
- [ ] 6
- [ ] E

COMMENTS: *General anesthesia discussed along with risks/benefits. Questions answered.*

MISCELLANEOUS
- [ ] pregnancy
- [ ] malnutrition
- [ ] weight loss
- [ ] deafness
- [ ] glaucoma
- [ ]
- [ ] obesity
- [ ] substance abuse *NONE*
- [ ] alcohol ~~abuse~~ *NONE*
- [ ] other _____

HEPATIC / G.I. *Denies Sx GE reflux*
- [ ] hepatitis
- [ ] jaundice
- [ ] hiatal hernia
- [ ] other _____

HEMATOLOGIC
Denies anemia, bleeding tendencies

RENAL ∅
- [ ] dialysis
- [ ] failure
- [ ] other _____

ENDOCRINE ∅
- [ ] diabetes
- [ ] hyperthyroid
- [ ] hypothyroid
- [ ] other _____

ADVERSE REACTIONS / ALLERGIES
PCN / SULFA → RASH
Denies latex or iodine sensitivities

MEDICATIONS / MEDICAL APPLIANCES
Estrogen supplementation - DC'd 10-13

LAB / X-RAY / ECG *NSR (70)*
- [ ] normal
- [ ] other _____ *Labs pending @ PDA visit*

DENTITION *Several gold crowns/fillings No partial chipped, cracked or loose teeth*
- [x] satisfactory
- [ ] other _____

Height *5'6½"* Weight *167#* NPO *p̄ MN instructed*

INFO / CONSENTS TO:
- [x] general
- [x] regional
- [ ] spinal
- [ ] epidural
- [ ] MAC

Signature: _____   Date *10-22-* *GFMA*

PRE-ANESTHESIC EVALUATION

05300230

05300230

FIGURE 5.26 Pre- and postanesthesia evaluation.

_____ Medical Center

ANESTHESIA DEPARTMENT

POST ANESTHESIA EVALUATION	POST ANESTHESIA COMPLICATIONS
VITAL SIGNS: ☐ Blood Pressure _____ ☐ Pulse _____ ☐ Respirations _____	**1. IMMEDIATE POST-OP DEATH**
	2. UNANTICIPATED ICU ADMISSION
THE PATIENT IS ☐ Awake ☑ Responding ☐ Alert ☑ Orientated	**3. CARDIOVASCULAR** ☐ M.I. ☐ angina ☐ C.H.F. ☐ arrythmias ☐ hypo / hypertension ☐ arrest
STATUS ☑ Satisfactory ☐ other _____	**4. PULMONARY** ☐ reintubation ☐ aspiration ☐ other _____
COMMENTS: _____ _____ _____ _____ _____ _____ _____	**5. ACUTE NEUROLOGIC** _____ _____
	6. INJURY ☐ eye ☐ dental ☐ other _____
	7. UNANTICIPATED INPATIENT ADMISSION OF A.S.C. PATIENT.

Signature: _____

Date _____   Time: _____

POST-ANESTHESIA EVALUATION / COMPLICATIONS   05300230

```
* 0 5 3 0 0 2 3 0 *
```

FIGURE 5.27 Postanesthesia evaluation.

CHART COPY

MEDICAL CENTER

ANESTHESIA RECORD

OPERATION PERFORMED	Axillary node	ANESTHESIA TYPE	DATE
ⓇSegmental Mastectomy - Diss		GA	10/24/

SURGEON/RESIDENT   DURATION OF OPERATION

ANESTHESIOLOGIST / CRNA   DURATION OF ANESTHESIA

C S   MR
M02.805 SCE
05/12/3?   60   F   1575

ENDOTRACHEAL:
SIZE 7.5 BLADE 11 LTA Y N
ORO ___ NASO R L CUFF ___

AGENTS-TECHNIQUES

AGE < 1 > 70
FIELD
AVOID

NASAL/ORAL AIRWAY/N. CANNULA Y N
REMARKS _____

MACHINE CHECK ☑
O₂ FLOW ☐   SPARE ☐
POWER ☐   TANKS ☐
SUCTION ☐   PRESS ☐
MONITOR ☑   LEAKS ☑

APGAR:
1 min ___
5 min ___

PHYSICAL STATUS: (ASA)
1 2 ③ 4 5 6 E

AGENTS

Thiopen	15	
Sch ai	100	
Pavulon	4	
L/min. N₂O/AIR		
L/min. O₂	6	2
INH-AGENT		
Sevofl	1	D.7-09-07-10

REMARKS

Glyco 0.2 mg
Zofran 4 mg
Propofol .0 mg
Pos 3.0 mg
Erythromycin
500 mg 1455
1445 M. Roli relief
1520 Neostigmine 3mg / Robinul 0.9

O₂% SAT	250	
ETPCO₂		
URINE		
TEMP.		
	200	
C.V.P.		
P.A.		
P.C.W.P.	150	
C.O.		
● PULSE		
O RESP	100	
V B.P.		
X ANES.		
O OPER.	50	
T TOURN.		
▲ B.L. GAS		
V VENTIL	0	

FOR REMARKS

TRAIN OF 4   4/4

EKG

POSITION   0-1

MONITORING

STEPH P/E	PULSE OX	BL. WARM
E.K.G.	VENT./SERVO	ART. LINE
N.B.P.	MASS SP.	CVP/PA
TEMP.	FOLEY	DOPPLER
O₂ MON.	N.G. TUBE	FIBEROPTIC
T OF 4	BLANKET	JACK/REESE

P.R.B.C.	
F.F.P.	
W.B.	
P.L.T.	
ALBUMIN	
TOTAL	

CRYSTOLLOIDS

5% DLR	1000	500
LR	1000	500
0.9 NaCl	1000	500
5% D/.2NS	1000	500
5% D/.45NS	1000	500
5% D/H₂O	1000	500

INTAKE
TOTAL

I.V. SITE	I.V. SIZE	TIME
		FIO₂
		pH
		pCO₂
		pO₂
		HCO₂
		BE
		O₂ SAT
		HGB
		HCT
		K

PAR
ICU
UNIT
ARA

TIME TRANSFERRED   BP ___ mmHg   PULSE ___ /min   RESP ___ /min

(NON) RESPONSIVE   STABLE   SIGNATURE

OUTPUT URINE _____
TOTAL   BLOOD _____

05100120 2-97

FIGURE 5.28 Anesthesia record.

MEDICAL CENTER

ANESTHESIA RECORD

CHART COPY

OPERATION PERFORMED		ANESTHESIA TYPE	DATE
SURGEON/RESIDENT	DURATION OF OPERATION		
ANESTHESIOLOGIST / CRNA	DURATION OF ANESTHESIA		

```
CS            MR
         M02,B05 SCE
                      1575
CS/10/37   60      F
```

ENDOTRACHEAL:

SIZE _____ BLADE _____ LTA Y N
ORO _____ NASO _R_ _L_ CUFF _____

NASAL/ORAL AIRWAY/N. CANNULA _Y N_
REMARKS _____

AGENTS-TECHNIQUES		AGE <1 >70 FIELD AVOID

MACHINE CHECK ☐
O₂ FLOW ☐   SPARE ☐
POWER ☐   TANKS ☐
SUCTION ☐   PRESS ☐
MONITOR ☐   LEAKS ☐

APGAR:
1 min ___
5 min ___

PHYSICAL STATUS: (ASA)
1 2 3 4 5 6 E _____

AGENTS															REMARKS

L/min. N2O/AIR   5 — 8
L/min. O₂   2 — 6
INH-AGENT   1 — K

		MONITORING		
STEPH P/E	PULSE OX	BL. WARM
E.K.G.	VENT./SERVO	ART. LINE
N.B.P.	MASS SP.	CVP/PA
TEMP.	FOLEY	DOPPLER
O₂ MON.	N.G. TUBE	FIBEROPTIC
T OF 4	BLANKET	JACK/REESE

O₂% SAT — 250
ETPCO₂
URINE
TEMP. — 200
C.V.P.
P.A.
P.C.W.P. — 150
C.O.
● PULSE
O RESP — 100
V B.P.
X ANES.
⊙ OPER. — 50
T TOURN.
▲ B.L. GAS
V VENTIL — 0
FOR REMARKS
TRAIN OF 4
EKG
POSITION

P.R.B.C.	
F.F.P.	
W.B.	
P.L.T.	
ALBUMIN	
TOTAL	

I.V. SITE	I.V. SIZE	TIME	
		FIO₂	
		pH	
		pCO₂	
		pO₂	
		HCO₃	
		BE	
		O₂ SAT	
		HGB	
		HCT	
		K	

	CRYSTOLLOIDS	
5% DLR	1000	500
LR	1000	500
0.9 NaCl	1000	500
5% D/.2NS	1000	500
5% D/.45NS	1000	500
5% D/H₂O	1000	500

INTAKE
TOTAL   900 cc

PAR	TIME	1800	BP 16 21/10 mmHg	PULSE 113 /min	RESP 20 /min
ICU	TRANSFERRED				
UNIT	(NON) RESPONSIVE STABLE		SIGNATURE		
ARA					

OUTPUT
TOTAL
URINE _____
BLOOD _200 cc_

05100120 2-97

FIGURE 5.28 Continued.

OR NURSING RECORD

PREOPERATIVE STATUS   ☐ OR   ☑ Holding Area   Time 1325   Date 10/24/

	Yes	No	LEVEL OF CONSCIOUS	SKIN CONDITION
Permit	☑	☐	☑ Oriented ☐ Semiconscious	☑ Warm ☐ Pale
H&P	☑	☐	☐ Confused ☐ Apprehensive	☐ Cool ☐ Pink
Lab	☑	☐	☐ Agitated ☐ Comatose	☑ Dry ☐ Flushed
XRay	☑	☐	☑ Relaxed ☐ Restrained	☐ Diaphoretic
EKG	☑	☐		

Allergies ☑ ☐ Sulfa, Penn PCN
~~Error~~

DRAINS, TUBES, IV'S ☑ None   **BLOOD** _____
☐ IV ☐ Foley ☐ Chest ☐ NG   **SIGNATURE:**
☐ Other _____

☐ Inpatient   ☑ Outpatient

OS   MR
          MO2,805 SCE
                     157
05/10/37   60   F

INTRAOPERATIVE CARE	OR ROOM #	OR ARRIVAL	OP START	OP END	OUT OF ROOM
	2	1335	1400	1745	1755

PROCEDURE: Right segmental mastectomy and axillary Dissection

PREOP DIAGNOSIS: Carcinoma right breast

POSTOP DIAGNOSIS: same

Surgeon:	2nd Assist: JMS	
1st Assist: MD	3rd Assist: /	
Anesthetic: General	Anesthetic By: RE	
Anesthetic Tech:	Anesthetic Res:	
Circulator:	Relieved By: STP 1500 - ~~End~~ 1700	
Scrub:	Relieved By: PB 1700 - END	
Med Nurse:	Relieved By:	
Pump Tech:	Balloon Tech:	

WOUND CLASS/TECH BREAKS ☑ None
① 2 3   ☐ Yes   See Nursing Notes

DRAINS	COUNTS ☐ N/A
☐ NONE	1st Count Circ STP/PB Scrub RD/KD
☐ Hemovac	2nd Count Circ STP/PB Scrub RD/KD
☐ Penrose	☑ Sponges ☑ Needles ☑ Instruments
☐ Duvall	Count ☑ Correct
☑ J-Vac	☐ Incorrect See Nsg Notes
☐ Other	☐ Terminal Xray

DRESSING / PACKINGS ¼" Steri-Strips
☐ None fluffs

MEDICATIONS / IRRIGATIONS
Lymphazurin 5cc

NURSES NOTES Patient stated understanding of procedure. Warm blankets for comfort. Reaction & kells ___ ___ Arrow medical supply rep in room throughout case. 15 FR Round DRAIN to GRENADE RESERVOIR

SAFETY MEASURES	Yes	No
Table locked	☑	☐
Safety belt	☑	☐
If no why _____		
Padding applied	☑	☐
If yes see Nsg notes		
Armboards	R ☑ L ☑	
Arms Tucked	R ☐ L ☐	

ESU #1   Yes ☐ No ☑
Serial # R4C4563-5
Location L thigh
Skin Cond. after Removal
☑ Intact
☐ Other: See Nsg Notes

ESU #2   Yes ☐ No ☑
Serial # _____
Location _____
Skin Cond. after Removal
☐ Intact
☐ Other: See Nsg Notes

FOLEY CATHETER ☑ None
☐ Straight ☐ Indwelling
____Fr ____Balloon
Return ____ cc's
Removed · Yes ☐ No ☐
Inserted by _____

PREP AREA/TYPE	R	L
☐ Heart ☐ Arm	☐ ☐	
☐ Abdomen ☐ Leg	☐ ☐	
☐ Perineal ☑ Breast	☑ ☑	
☐ Cranial ☐ Eye	☐ ☐	
☐ Facial ☐ Ear	☐ ☐	
☐ Back ☐ Chest	☐ ☐	
☐ Other		

PREP SOLUTION ☐ None
☑ Betadine ☐ Duraprep
☐ Hibiclens ☐ Other
By: RV

PT POSITION
☑ Supine
☐ Lithotomy ☐ Frog legged
☐ Prone ☐ Lateral
☐ Fowlers ☐ R ☐ L
☐ Other _____

POSITIONING AIDS ☑ None
☐ Olympic bag ☐ Footrolls
☐ Wilson frame ☐ Sandbag
☐ Prone Armboard ☐ Stirrups

CELL SAVER Yes ☐ No ☑
Amount _____
THERMIA UNIT # ____ By: ____
Time Bair hugger Temp

TOURNIQUET ☑ None
Unit # _____
Tested by _____

☐ Arm ☐ R ☐ Arm ☐ R
☐ Leg ☐ L ☐ Leg ☐ L

Up _____
Down _____
Press _____

LASER Yes ☐ No ☑
☐ CO$_2$ Other _____
Mode _____ Wattage _____

XRAY Yes ☐ No ☑
☐ Regular ☐ Image
Site _____

IMPLANTS ☑ None
☐ Documented in progress notes.
☐ Documented on OR record

SPECIMENS TO LAB
Specimens ☑ Yes # 6 ☐ No
Frozen ☑ Yes # 1 ☐ No
Cultures ☐ Yes # ___ ☐ No

LOCAL MONITORING NA

Time				
BP				
Pulse				
Time				
BP				
Pulse				

Patient Transfer to: ☐ Outpatient ☐ CVICU ☐ Floor
☐ Other _____ ☒ Recovery ☐ ICU Room # ___

Method of Transfer: ☒ Cart ☐ Bed ☐ W/C ☐ Walk
POST OP STATUS REPORT TO PAR EXTUBATED

NAME	INITIALS	NAME	INITIALS	NAME	INITIALS
RV	RV		STP		
OCT	KD		PB		

Medical Center   05205713

FIGURE 5.29 OR clinical record.

—461—

POST ANESTHESIA CARE UNIT RECORD — PACU form

ADMISSION DATE & TIME	SURGEON	ANESTHESIOLOGIST
10/24 C1800		

TYPE OF ANESTHESIA: ☒ GENERAL ☐ SPINAL ☐ MAC ☐ CAUDAL ☐ EPIDURAL ☐ BLOCK ☐ Other:

AIRWAY: ☐ ORAL ☐ NASAL ☐ ENDOTRACHEAL
☒ NATURAL   DC Time___   DC Time___   DC Time___

☐ Ventilator Mode

OXYGEN: ☐ Tube ___% ___L/Min. ☒ Mask ___L/Min. On 1800 Off 1830 ☒ Cannula ___L/Min. On 1845 Off cont. ☐ Puritan ___% ___L/Min. ☐ None ___On ___Off

___ F₁O₂ ___ VT ___ Rate ___ On ___ Off

PROCEDURE: Right Segmental Mastectomy and Right axillary lymph node dissection

Pre-Op BP: 177/85 p.88

EKG Rhythm: sinus

APPEARANCE: ☐ Pale ☒ Pink ☐ Jaundiced ☐ Cyanotic ☐ Shivering ☐ Other___

CONDITION OF SKIN: ☒ Dry ☐ Moist ☐ Warm ☐ Cool ☐ Other___

DRAINS: ☐ N/A ☐ FOLEY___ ☐ CBI___ ☐ NG___ ☒ WOUND DRAIN ___ ☐ OTHER___

DRESSING: ☐ N/A LOCATION Right breast side c ___

☐ PACKING ☐ PENROSE___ ☐ OTHER___

ORTHOPEDIC ASSESSMENT: ☒ N/A ☐ CAST ☐ WET ☐ ICE ☐ ELEVATION ☐ ACE ☐ DRY ☐ OTHER___ LOCATION___

GRAPHIC KEY
- ⋎ – Dynamap
- x / x – A Line
- • – Pulse

ASSESSMENTS
- ↙ – No Significant Finding
- ∗ – See Notes Status unchanged

Time					
220					
200					
180					
160					
140					
120					
100					
80					
60					
40					

RESPIRATIONS	20	20	20	20	20
SWAN/CVP					
PULSE OXIMETRY	98	98	96	98	98
TEMPERATURE	95			97	

PACU SCORE

ACTIVITY voluntary or by command 2 = Moves 4 extremities 1 = Moves 2 extremities 0 = Moves 0 extremities	2	2	2	2	2
RESPIRATION 2 = Able to deep breathe / cough 1 = Dyspnea / Limited 0 = Apnea	2	2	2	2	
CIRCULATION 2 = BP ± 20% of pre-op. 1 = BP ± 20-50% of pre-op. 0 = BP ± 50% of pre-op.	2	2	2	2	
CONSCIOUSNESS 2 = Awake 1 = Arousable 0 = Unresponsive	1	2	2	2	
COLOR 2 = Normal skin color 1 = Pale, blotchy, other 0 = Cyanotic, dusky	2	2	2	2	
TOTALS	9	10	10	10	10
RESPIRATORY ASSESSMENT	✓				
NEUROLOGICAL ASSESSMENT	✓				
CARDIOVASCULAR ASSESSMENT	✓				
SURGICAL SITE ASSESSMENT	✓	✓	✓	✓	
TUBE ASSESSMENT	✓	✓	✓	✓	
PAIN ASSESSMENT / RATING					
NEUROVASCULAR ASSESSMENT	✓	✓	✓	✓	
URINARY ASSESSMENT					
GASTROINTESTINAL ASSESS.					
R. N. INITIALS					

MEDICATIONS

Time	Medication	Dose	Route
1820	Demerol 50 mg		IM

POST ANESTHESIA CARE UNIT RECORD X4480   Medical Center

FIGURE 5.30 Postanesthesia care unit record and care plan.

PATIENT PROGESS NOTE (Nurses Note)

TIME	FOCUS	

Time					
hgb					
hct					
Ph					
PCO$_2$					
PO$_2$					
HCO$_3$					
O$_2$ SAT					
NA					
K					
cl					
CO$_2$					
GLU					

MISCELLANEOUS:

CVP / SWAN SITE:

INTAKE: IV Solution

Time	Site	Solution	cc/in	cc/left
1800	Rhd	1000cc LR	100	
		D5.45NaCl —		→1000

TOTAL IV	100	1000cc
TOTAL IRRIGATION		
TOTAL BLOOD/ PRODUCTS		
TOTAL INTAKE	(100)	

OUTPUT

Time	Foley	Hemovac	NG	Void	Other
TOTAL					

TOTAL OUTPUT (0)

FOCUS LIST:

- ☒ Airway Management
- ☒ Comfort
- ☐ Thermoregulation
- ☐ Thought process
- ☐ Communication
- ☐ Knowledge Deficit
- ☐ Hemodynamic
- ☐ Nausea Vomiting
- ☐ Other

UNRESOLVED FOCI:

- ☒
- ☐
- ☐
- ☐
- ☐
- ☐
- ☐
- ☐
- ☐

Communication of Abnormal Assessment:

Patient transferred: 4 North.   By: Carl   Condition: ☒ Stable   ☐ Unstable

Report given to: RN

Discharge Time: 1900

Admission RN RH   **Relief RN**   **Discharge RN** M

Acuity Level   1   2   3   4   ☒ Care delivered as per Standards/Policy Procedure

X4480

FIGURE 5.30 Continued.

PACU STANDARDIZED FOCUS CARE PLAN

FOCUS STATEMENT: Airway Management

Time Implemented __1842__

PATIENT DATA: *(check appropriate box and/or add individualized one)*

☐ 1. Muscle relaxants/anesthetic agents
☐ 2. Type of surgical procedure
☐ 3. Dysrythmias
☐ 4. Dependance on artificial airway
☐ 5. Partial airway obstruction with adequate gas exchange
☐ 6. Partial airway obstruction with inadequate gas exchange
☐ 7. Complete airway obstruction
☒ 8. Low oxygen saturation with patent airway
☐ 9. Other: *(specify)*

NURSING ACTIONS: *(check appropriate box and/or add individualized one)*

☐ 1. Assess respiratory rate, quality and exchange upon admission, every 15 minutes during patient's stay and PRN.
☐ 2. Provide/maintain airway support as needed
   ☐ Jaw support   ☐ Insertion of airways   ☐ Ventilator   ☐ ETT
   ☐ Stir up regime   ☐ Ambu assist   ☐ Nasal/Oral
☐ 3. Suction as needed
   ☐ a. ETT
   ☐ b. Nasal
   ☐ c. Oral
☐ 4. Removal of ETT when criteria is met
☐ 5. Assist with reintubation as needed
☐ 6. Monitor ABG's PRN
☒ 7. Pulse oximetry
☐ 8. Other: *(specify)*

PATIENT RESPONSE: *(check appropriate box)*

☐ 1. Resolved, patient returned to pre-op baseline
☒ 2. Unresolved, to be followed through on receiving unit.
☒ 3. O₂ Continued on receiving unit per orders.

TARGET DATE: *(check appropriate box)*

☒ 1. Upon discharge from PACU

Date: __10/24__   Time: __19³⁰__

Nurses Signature: _____

X4488 (Rev. 11/94) - 56

PACU STANDARDIZED FOCUS CARE PLAN

FOCUS STATEMENT: Thought Process

Time Implemented _____

PATIENT DATA: *(check appropriate box and/or add individualized one)*

☐ 1. Anesthesia
☐ 2. Adverse reaction to Ketamine
☐ 3. IV sedation
☐ 4. Response to severe pain
☐ 5. Anoxia
☐ 6. Disorientation to time, place, person, events
☐ 7. Restlessness
☐ 8. Other: *(specify)*

NURSING ACTIONS: *(check appropriate box and/or add individualized one)*

☐ 1. Assess LOC upon admission, every 15 minutes and PRN.
☐ 2. Orient patient to person, place, and time.
☐ 3. Allow children to wake up slowly.
☐ 4. Protect from injury PRN
☐ 5. Other: *(specify)*

PATIENT RESPONSE: *(check appropriate box)*

☐ 1. Resolved, patient returned to pre-op baseline
☐ 2. Unresolved, to be followed through on receiving unit.

TARGET DATE:

☐ 1. Upon discharge from PACU

Date: _____   Time: _____

Nurses Signature: _____

FIGURE 5.30 Continued.

PACU STANDARDIZED FOCUS CARE PLAN

FOCUS STATEMENT: Comfort

Time Implemented _1820_

PATIENT DATA: *(check appropriate box and/or add individualized one)*

- [ ] 1. Psychological or physical response to surgical procedure.
- [ ] 2. Ineffectiveness of intra operative analgesic.
- [x] 3. Subjective
  - [x] a. verbal communication of quality/location _"leg hurting"_
  - [ ] b. type of pain scale used _Numerical_
  - [ ] c. pain scale designation _8_
- [ ] 4. Objective
  - [ ] a. guarding behavior
  - [ ] b. distractive behavior (moaning, crying, restlessness).
  - [ ] c. facial masking of pain
  - [ ] d. autonomic response (diaphoresis, BP, or P change, change in respirations, or pupillary dilation)
  - [ ] e. Other: *(specify)* _____

NURSING ACTIONS: *(check appropriate box and/or add individualized one)*

- [ ] 1. Assess physiological/psychological response to pain upon admission, every 30 minutes and PRN.
- [x] 2. Assess verbal indicators of pain utilizing the pain scale, upon admission, when possible, every 30 minutes and PRN
- [x] 3. Administer analgesics _as per directive_
- [ ] 4. Provide comfort and/or distractive measures PRN.
  - [ ] a. ice packs
  - [ ] b. elevate extremity R _____ L _____
  - [x] c. apply warm blankets
  - [ ] d. relaxation exercises
  - [ ] Other: *(specify)* _____

PATIENT RESPONSE: *(check appropriate box)*

- [x] 1. Resolved - obtained post operative pain relief per pain scale _____
- [ ] 2. Unresolved - to be followed through on floor per pain scale _____

TARGET DATE:

- [x] 1. Upon discharge from PACU

Date: _10/23_   Time: _19 00_

Nurses Signature: _RN_

X4488

PACU STANDARDIZED FOCUS CARE PLAN

FOCUS STATEMENT: Nausea/Vomiting

Time Implemented _____

PATIENT DATA: *(check appropriate box and/or add individualized one)*

- [ ] 1. Anesthesia
- [ ] 2. Narcotics
- [ ] 3. Cardiac Glycosides
- [ ] 4. C/O queasiness, urge to vomit.
- [ ] 5. Flushed
- [ ] 6. Pallor
- [ ] 7. Diaphoresis
- [ ] 8. Other: *(specify)* _____

NURSING ACTIONS: *(check appropriate box and/or add individualized one)*

- [ ] 1. Assess for any evidence of N/V every 15 minutes during PACU stay, and prn.
- [ ] 2. Protect patient from aspiration.
- [ ] 3. Administer antiemetics.
- [ ] 4. Other: *(specify)* _____

PATIENT RESPONSE: *(check appropriate box)*

- [ ] 1. Resolved - obtained relief from nausea
- [ ] 2. Unresolved - to be followed through on receiving unit.

TARGET DATE:

- [ ] 1. Upon discharge from PACU

Date: _____   Time: _____

Nurses Signature: _____

FIGURE 5.30 Continued.

Medical Center

DS ¹⁰²⁴   MR
              M02,805 SCE
05/10/37 60   F   1575

PRE-PROCEDURE CHECKLIST

For the minimum pre-surgery and pre-procedure requirements and for general guidelines, see the reverse side of form.
Items with an "**S**" are to be completed on surgery patients with anesthesia involvement. Items with a "*****" are to be completed on surgery patients with local or no anesthesia involvement. Items with a "**C**" are to be completed on patients going for Cath Lab or E. Phys.

PRE-PROCEDURE CHECKLIST	Date	Initials	Comments
SC* 1. Allergies:	10·24	KL	penicillin sulfa
SC* 2. Pre-Procedure: Height _008_ m. Weight _76·1_ kgs./_167.5_ lbs.	✓		
SC* 3. Pre-Procedure teaching completed and documented	✓		
SC* 4. General hospital consent signed			
SC* 5. Procedure consent(s) signed	10·24	KL	
SC* 6. Physician's pre-procedure orders checked and completed			
SC 7. History and physical on chart			
SC 8. Chest X-ray too holding			
SC ✓9. EKG			
SC 10 Lab work completed as ordered and on chart			
SC 11 Hgb___ Hct___ K+___ Creatinine___ BUN___ PT___ PTT___			
✓12 Urinalysis results on chart	✓	↳	
SC* 13 Pregnancy test results on chart			
SC 14 Type and screen / cross # of units___ Blood Band #___			
SC 15 NPO after _____ 2400	10·24	KL	
S 16 Skin prep completed			
S 17 Bowel prep completed			
C 18 Pulses marked			
SC 19 Old records to unit / surgery			
TO BE CHECKED ON ALL PATIENTS 1-2 HOURS PRE-PROCEDURE			
20 ID, Blood, Allergy bands on	10·24	K	
21 Hospital gown on	✓	✓	
22 ☑ TEDS / SCDS thigh ☐ NG Tube inserted	10·24	KL	
23 ☐ Patient voided ( ) Time___			
24 ☐ IV started: Date___ Gauge___ Location___			
25 ITEMS REMOVED: ☐ Dentures ☐ Removable Bridge			
☐ Contact Lenses ☐ Glasses ☐ Hearing Aid			
☐ Prosthesis ☐ Hairpins ☐ Wigs & Hairpieces			
☑ Personal Clothing ☐ Make-up ☐ Nail Polish ☐ Jewelry	10·24	KL	
Note what items are sent with patient ___			
26 Vital signs: Time_0830_ BP_111/85_ Pulse_88_ Resp_20_ PO₂_96_ Temp_97.6_	10·24	KL	
27 Pre-procedure medications given and charted			
28 Medications to be administered: ☐ Attached to chart ☐ Sent directly to procedure unit			
29 Addressograph plate / labels on chart	10·24	KL	
30 Patient data form on chart			
31 IV profile in chart			
32 Medication Administration Record on chart			

TO: _Ultrasound_

Date: _10·24-_   MODE: CONDITION:
Time: _0845_   ☐ Cart   ☐ Stable
                 ☑ W/C   ☐ Other (See notes)
                 ☐ Ambulatory
Sending RN: _____ RN

RECEIVED IN: _HA_

Date: _10/24/_   MODE: CONDITION:
Time: _1325_   ☐ Cart   ☑ Stable
                 ☑ W/C   ☐ Other (See notes)
                 ☐ Ambulatory
Receiving RN: _____

05100760

05100760

FIGURE 5.31 Preoperative checklist.

Medical Center

IV THERAPY PROFILE
05200620 (Rev. 1/95) - 70

NAME: _____

ROOM: _____

Start Date R.Ph/RN	IV SOLUTIONS Base Solution / Blood Product	Additives	Volume (ml)	Rate	Stop Date R.Ph/RN	Date	Date	Date	Date	Date
10/24	5D .45 NaCl		1000cc	1000/hr.	Date 10/24 1500	10/25				
10/24	D5 .45 NS	—	1000c	1000cc%		M9540				

FIGURE 5.32 Medication administration record.

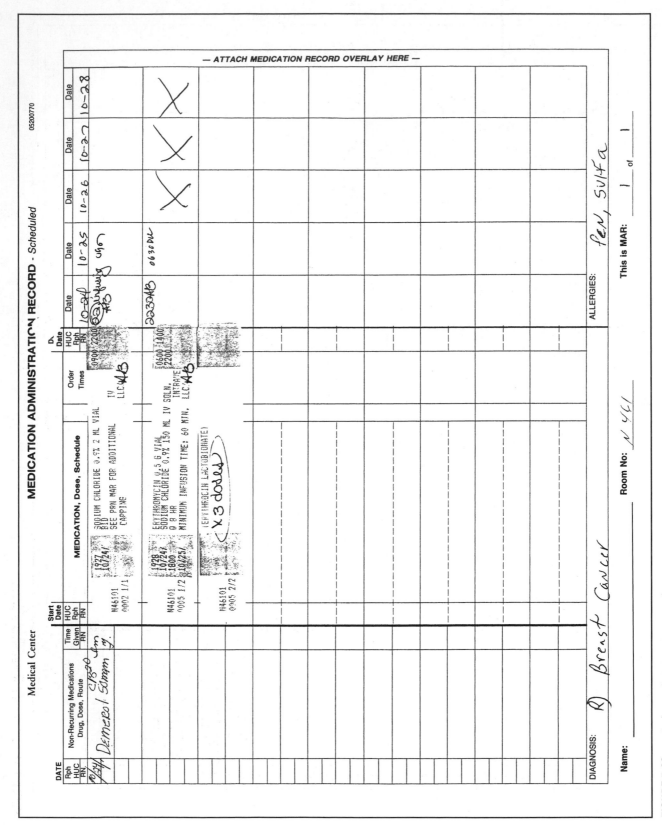

FIGURE 5.33 Medication administration record.

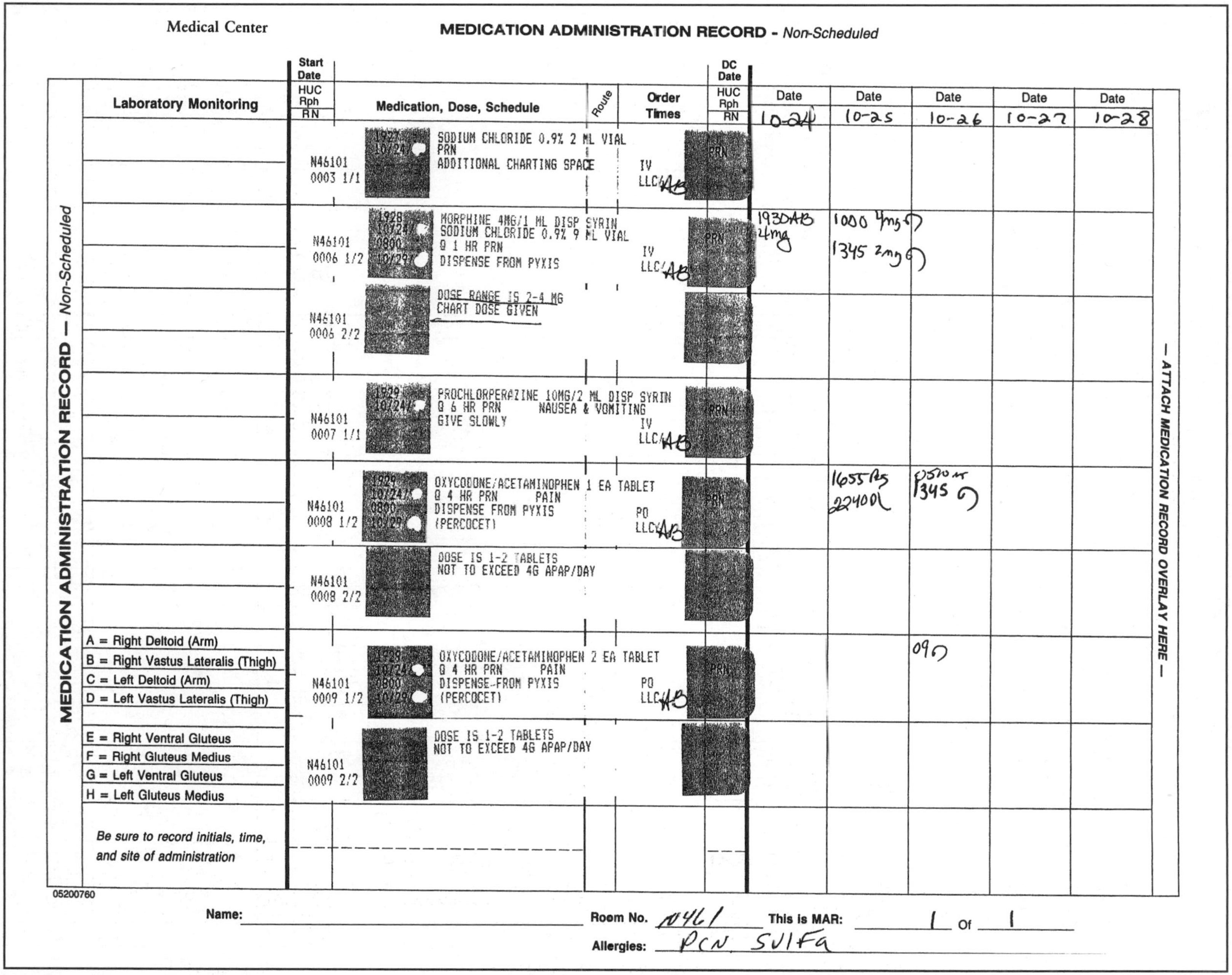

Medical Center

MEDICATION ADMINISTRATION RECORD - *Non-Scheduled*

Laboratory Monitoring	Start Date HUC Rph RN	Medication, Dose, Schedule	Route	Order Times	DC Date HUC Rph RN	Date 10-24	Date 10-25	Date 10-26	Date 10-27	Date 10-28
	N46101 0003 1/1	SODIUM CHLORIDE 0.9% 2 ML VIAL PRN ADDITIONAL CHARTING SPACE	IV	LLC/AB	PRN					
	N46101 0006 1/2	MORPHINE 4MG/1 ML DISP SYRIN SODIUM CHLORIDE 0.9% 9 ML VIAL Q 1 HR PRN DISPENSE FROM PYXIS	IV	LLC/AB	PRN	1930 AB 4mg	1000 4mg; 1345 2mg			
	N46101 0006 2/2	DOSE RANGE IS 2-4 MG CHART DOSE GIVEN								
	N46101 0007 1/1	PROCHLORPERAZINE 10MG/2 ML DISP SYRIN Q 6 HR PRN NAUSEA & VOMITING GIVE SLOWLY	IV	LLC/AB	PRN					
	N46101 0008 1/2	OXYCODONE/ACETAMINOPHEN 1 EA TABLET Q 4 HR PRN PAIN DISPENSE FROM PYXIS (PERCOCET)	PO	LLC/AB	PRN		1655 RS; 2240	0510; 1345		
	N46101 0008 2/2	DOSE IS 1-2 TABLETS NOT TO EXCEED 4G APAP/DAY								
A = Right Deltoid (Arm) B = Right Vastus Lateralis (Thigh) C = Left Deltoid (Arm) D = Left Vastus Lateralis (Thigh)	N46101 0009 1/2	OXYCODONE/ACETAMINOPHEN 2 EA TABLET Q 4 HR PRN PAIN DISPENSE-FROM PYXIS (PERCOCET)	PO	LLC/AB	PRN			09		
E = Right Ventral Gluteus F = Right Gluteus Medius G = Left Ventral Gluteus H = Left Gluteus Medius	N46101 0009 2/2	DOSE IS 1-2 TABLETS NOT TO EXCEED 4G APAP/DAY								
Be sure to record initials, time, and site of administration										

— ATTACH MEDICATION RECORD OVERLAY HERE —

MEDICATION ADMINISTRATION RECORD — Non-Scheduled

05200760

Name: ______ Room No. N461 This is MAR: 1 Of 1

Allergies: PCN Sulfa

FIGURE 5.34 Medication administration record.

NURSING DATA BASE / DISCHARGE PLAN

Locker #17

ADMISSION STATUS 30 Day re-admit: ☐ NO ☐ YES

Date: ____ Time of admission ____

PATIENT HAS BEEN INFORMED:
- ☒ Room lights
- ☒ Phone/TV service
- ☒ Religious services
- ☒ Non-smoking policy
- ☒ Emergency lights
- ☒ Security for valuables
- ☒ Visiting hours
- ☒ Nurse call
- ☒ Bed control operation

Initials: ____

PATIENT / SIGNIFICANT OTHER UNDERSTANDING OF REASON FOR HOSPITALIZATION?

VITAL SIGNS
PREADMISSION ____ Initials ____
(DATE: ____) T ____ P ____ R ____ BP ____ L ____ R ____
Height ____ Weight ____ #
ADMISSION ____ Initials ____
(DATE: ____) T ____ P ____ R ____ BP ____ L ____ R ____
Height ____ Weight ____ Weight ____

DOES PATIENT HAVE AN ADVANCE DIRECTIVE?
- ☐ No, information given to patient / S.O
- ☐ Yes, advance directive copy on chart
- ☐ Unknown
Date ____

HAS PATIENT SIGNED AN ORGAN DONOR CARD?
- ☐ Yes,
- ☐ No,
Date ____

MR
M02, R05   SCE
1575
05-13-37   60 F

PREVIOUS SURGERIES / INJURIES

ALLERGIES / SENSITIVITIES (SPECIFY MEDICATION OR SUBSTANCE)   **REACTIONS**
- ☒ Medication(s)   Penicillin — Hives
- ☒ Latex — denies
- ☒ Anesthesia — denies
- ☐ Other:

DOCTORS / NURSES YOU SEE

CLINICS YOU GO TO

HEALTH HISTORY
- ☐ High blood pressure
- ☐ Heart disease
- ☐ Heart palpitations / Skipped beats
- ☐ Rheumatic heart disease
- ☐ Stroke
- ☐ Fainting /Dizzy spells
- ☐ Seizure / Epilepsy
- ☒ Cancer
- ☒ Musculoskeletal problems
- ☒ Arthritis
- ☐ Lung disease
- ☐ History of or exposure to tuberculosis
- ☐ Stomach problems
- ☐ Bowel problems
- ☐ Diabetes
- ☐ Unexplained weight change ____ + ____ lbs. − ____ lbs.
- ☐ Liver disease
- ☐ Hepatitis
- ☐ Sickle Cell
- ☐ Bleeding problems
- ☐ Glaucoma
- ☒ Vision problems
- ☐ Hearing problems
- ☐ Urinary problems
- ☐ Kidney problems
- ☒ History of blood transfusion
- ☒ Alcohol / Drug abuse
- ☐ History of needle sharing
- ☐ History of unsafe sex
- ☐ Positive HIV
- ☐ Sexually transmitted disease
- ☐ History of sexual assault or abuse
- ☐ History of family violence
- ☐ Mental health problems
- ☐ Other.

Women: LMP date ____ Grav ____ Para (Term) ____ Preterm ____ Ab. ____ (Term) Ab. ____ Living ____
Last Pap Smear   date: ____
Last Mammogram   date: ____
☒ Practices self-breast examination − frequency ____
☐ GYN problems / Infertility

PRESCRIPTION MEDICATIONS Code: H - Home   B - Brought with patient   P - Pharmacy

Name of medication	Dose	How often	Why taking	Last time taken	Code

OVER THE COUNTER AND STREET DRUGS

Name of Drug	How often	Why taking	Last time taken	Code

Medical Center

05100900 -41(Rev. 8/95)

05100900

NURSING DATA BASE / DISCHARGE PLAN

FIGURE 5.35 Nursing database/discharge plan.

PERSONAL HEALTH HISTORY

Do you drink beer, wine or alcohol? ☒ No ☐ Yes How much? _____ Last drink? _____

Do you smoke? ☐ No ☐ Yes Amount/day? _____
Did you ever smoke? ☐ No ☒ Yes When did you stop? _10 yrs ago_
Are you on a special diet? ☐ No ☒ Yes (explain) _____
Are you worried about your health or hospitalization? ☒ No ☐ Yes (explain) _____
Coping mechanisms used _____

Do you have sleeping problems? ☒ No ☐ Yes (explain) _____
Do you exercise regularly? ☐ No ☒ Yes (explain) _walk 1 mi daily_

SOCIAL HISTORY

FAMILY HEALTH HISTORY

Family Composition
☒ Lives alone
☐ Spouse/partner
☐ Single parent
☐ Lives with friends
☐ Lives with extended family
☐ Has children (How many? _0_) (# living at home ____)
☐ Other (explain) _____

☐ Unknown
☒ Heart disease _dad ↓_
☒ Stroke _aunt ↓_
☐ High Blood Pressure
☐ Diabetes
☒ Cancer _mom (lives) m. uncles lives_
☐ Seizure/Epilepsy _↓ m. aunt_
Reaction to anesthesia _↓ m. aunt_
☐ Adopted
☐ Other (explain) _↑ bro prostate_

Occupation: (_retired American) momma_
Religious Preferences/Special Practices: _& will_

Cultural Needs ☒ No ☐ Yes (specify) _____

Family Spokesperson: _Catherine Arne_ PHONE: ( ) ___-___
_____ PHONE: ( ) ___-___
Guardian: _____ PHONE: ( ) ___-___

LEARNING NEEDS ASSESSMENT

Primary Language ☒ English ☐ Other (specify) _____

Able to
Speak English ☐ No ☒ Yes
Read English ☐ No ☒ Yes
Understand English ☐ No ☒ Yes
Sensory deficit ☒ No ☐ Yes (specify) _____

Preferred Method of Learning
☐ Reading
☐ Verbal instruction
☐ Demonstration
☐ Video/T.V.
☐ Other (specify) _____

Highest school grade completed: _college_

Significant other/support person to be included in patient teaching: _____

RN Signature _____ Date _N 10-33_ Time _____
(initiated)
05100900

DISCHARGE PLANNING

Admission Status
Admitted from ☒ Home ☐ Nursing Home

Type of assistance the patient received at home
☐ None   ☐ Transportation   ☐ Occupational therapy
☐ R.N.   ☐ Laundry   ☐ Physical therapy
☐ Nurse's aide   ☐ Housekeeping   ☐ Speech therapy
☐ Personal care ☐ Shopping   ☐ Other (specify)
☐ Meal preparation ☐ Medication administration

PROVIDER OF ASSISTANCE | TYPE OF SERVICE

Activities of Daily Living

	BATH	TOILET	DRESS/UNDRESS	TRANSFER	EATING	HOME	BROUGHT
Without help of any kind	✓	✓	✓	✓	✓		
Using assistive device(s)							
With help of another person							
Device and help of another person							
Other (explain)							

Assistive Devices	USES	HOME	BROUGHT		Assistive Devices	USES	HOME	BROUGHT
Crutches				Dentures	U L			
Cane				Partial	U L			
Walker				Contact Lenses	R L			
Wheelchair				Glasses (reading only distance)				(13)
Hospital bed				Oxygen				
Brace				Other (specify)				
Prosthesis								
Hearing Aid	R L							

Anticipated Need for Assistance with Home Health Maintenance
☐ Personal care   ☐ Skilled nursing   ☐ Cardiac rehab
☐ Housekeeping   ☐ Medication administration   ☐ Pulmonary service
☐ Meal preparation ☐ Patient/family teaching   ☐ Outpatient oncology
☐ Laundry   ☐ Occupational therapy   ☐ Financial assistance
☐ Shopping   ☐ Physical therapy   ☐ Other (explain)
☐ Transportation   ☐ Speech therapy

Plans for Living Arrangements
☒ Home ☐ Supervised Living ☐ Nursing Home ☐ Rehab

COMMENTS
Friends will stop in to help.
aunt and cousin will also help.

RN Signature _____ Date _____ Time _____
(completed)

FIGURE 5.35 Continued.

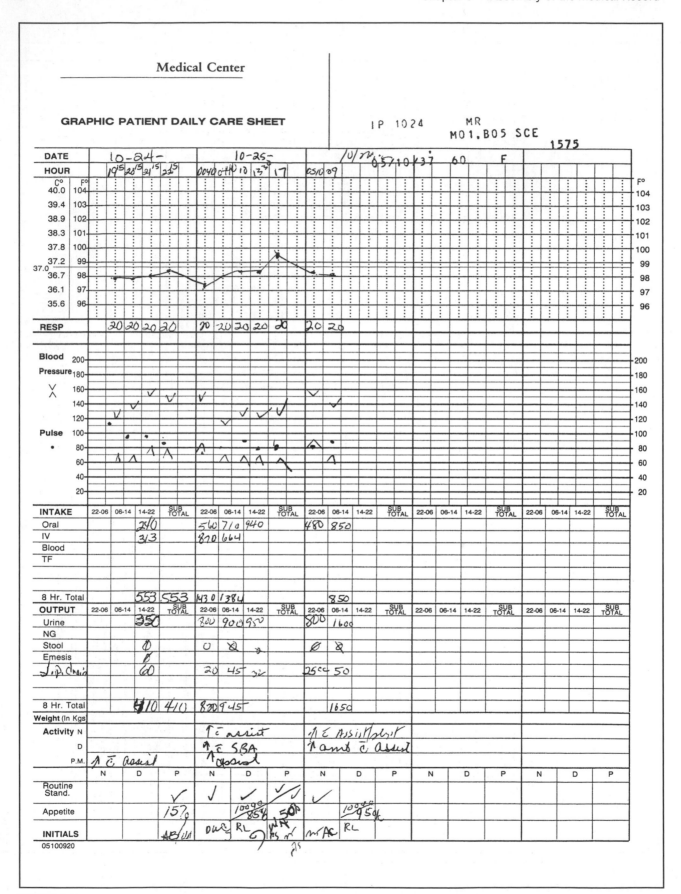

FIGURE 5.36 Graphic patient daily care sheet.

Medical Center

ASSESSMENT FLOW SHEET

```
IP 1024        MR
               M01,B05 SCE
                              1575
05/10/37   60   F
```

FOCUS	ORDERS	DATE	10-24	10-24	10-24	10-24	10-25	10-25	10/25	10/25	10/26	10/26	10/26	10/26
		TIME	1915	2015	2115	2215	0010	0500	0500	2135	0020	0370	0936	1030
POST-OP	Neurological		↑	↑	↓	↓	↓	↓	↓	↓	↓	·	↓	
(General)	Cardiovascular		✳	↓	↓	↓	↓	↓	↓	↓	↓		↓	
	Respiratory		↓	↑	↑	↑	↑	↑	✳	✳	→		↓	
	Surgical Dressing / Incision		↓	→/4	↑	↓	↓	↓	↓	↓	↓		↓	
	Pain Assessment / Rating		✳/10	→/5	→/4	→/4	→/3	→/4	6	7/4	7/2	7/4	2	✳
	G.U.		✳	↑	↑	✳	↑	↓	↓	↓	↓		↑	
	G.I.		✳	↑	↑	↑	↑	↑	✳	↑	↓		↓	
	Neurovascular		↓	↓	↓	↓	↓	↑	↑	↑	↑		↑	
	Musculoskeletal		✳	↑	↑	✳	↑	↓	↓	↓	↓		↓	
	Integumentary		↓	↓	↓	↓	↓	↓	↓	↓	↓		↓	
	Tubes: IV		↓	↓	↓	↓	↓	↓	↓	↓	↓		✳	✳
	JP drain													
	NURSE INITIAL →		AB	AB	AB	AB	DW	DW	DW	m	m	m	m	6

EQUIPMENT

TYPE	Initiate	D/C	TYPE	Initiate	D/C	TYPE	Initiate	D/C
Bladder Pump	10/04							

ASSESSMENT FLOW SHEET

See Reverse Side ▶

FIGURE 5.37 Assessment flow sheet.

GUIDELINES FOR USE OF THE ASSESSMENT FLOW SHEET

1. **FOCUS:** Indicate the Focus word or phrase in the focus column. The focus word connects the nursing orders to the specific nursing plan of care.

2. **ORDER:**

   a. Indicate the assessment/intervention order in the order column. The assessment/intervention orders coincide with the patient's plan of care. A physician order must be proceeded by M.O. in the orders column. If the nursing order includes one of the following standardized assessments, all the listed parameters must be assessed.

   "NEUROLOGICAL ASSESSMENT" — will include orientation, pupils, movement sensation, quality of speech and memory.

   "CARDIOVASCULAR ASSESSMENT" — will include apical pulse, neck veins, CRT, peripheral pulses, edema, and calf tenderness.

   "RESPIRATORY ASSESSMENT" — will include respiratory characteristics, breath sounds, cough, sputum, color of nailbeds / mucous membranes, and CRT.

   "GASTROINTESTINAL ASSESSMENT" — will include abdominal appearance, bowel sounds, palpation, diet tolerance, and stools.

   "GENITOURINARY ASSESSMENT" — will include voiding patterns, bladder distention, urine characteristics, or discharge.

   "INTEGUMENTARY ASSESSMENT" — will include skin color, skin temperature, skin integrity and condition of mucous membranes.

   "MUSCULOSKELETAL ASSESSMENT" — will include joint swelling, tenderness, limitations in ROM, muscle strength, and condition of surrounding tissue.

   "NEUROVASCULAR ASSESSMENT" — will include temperature, movement, CRT, peripheral pulses, edema, and patient description of sensation to affected extremity.

   "SURGICAL DRESSING / INCISIONAL ASSESSMENT" — will include condition of surgical dressing and/or color, temperature, tenderness of surrounding tissue, condition of sutures / staples / steri-strips, approximation of wound edges, and presence of any drainage.

   "PAIN ASSESSMENT" — will include patient description, location, duration, intensity, radiation, precipitating factors, and alleviating factors.

   "TUBE ASSESSMENT" — will include all invasive tubes / catheters including IVs, regarding patency, drainage, insertion site.

   "PSYCHO/SOCIAL ASSESSMENT" — will include appearance, behavior, communication patterns, orientation, memory, mood, and affect.

   "CHEMOTHERAPY ASSESSMENT" — will note the documentation for the delivery of any chemotherapy drugs.

   b. If the nurse chooses to modify the above standardized assessments, the modification must be noted on the plan of care.

   c. Assessments other than the standardized assessments must have defined assessment parameters and the expected findings on the plan of care.

3. **DATE / TIME:** The top of each column should be dated. Time of assessment should be indicated in the top of each small box.

4. **ORDER DOCUMENTATION SECTION:** Upon carrying out an order that has no significant findings, a "✓" in the appropriate category box is sufficient to indicate it was done. The following findings will be considered a negative assessment for the standardized parameters described above and constitute the use of a "✓".

   a. "NEUROLOGICAL ASSESSMENT" — Alert and oriented to person, place and time. Behavior appropriate to situation. Pupils equal and reactive to light. No headache or visual disturbances. Active ROM of all extremities with symmetry of strength. No paresthesia. Verbalization clear and understandable. Memory intact.

   b. "CARDIOVASCULAR ASSESSMENT" — Regular apical pulse. S₁ and S₂ audible. Neck veins flat at 45 degrees. CRT 3 seconds. Peripheral pulses palpable. No edema. No calf tenderness. No chest discomfort.

   c. "RESPIRATORY ASSESSMENT" — Respirations 12-20 / minute at rest. Respirations regular, quiet and easy without apparent effort. Breath sounds vesicular through both lung fields, bronchial over major airways. No adventitious sounds. Sputum clear. Nailbeds and mucous membranes pink. CRT < 3 seconds.

   d. "GASTROINTESTINAL ASSESSMENT" — Abdomen flat, soft, pliant musculature when relaxed; Active bowel sounds all 4 quadrants (5-34 minute). No visible or palpable masses. No pain with palpation. Tolerates diet without nausea or vomiting. Regular bowel pattern. No ostomies.

   e. "GENITOURINARY ASSESSMENT" — Urine clear and yellow to amber. No palpable bladder distension. No dysuria or frequency. No urethral or vaginal discharge. No catheter or ostomy.

   f. "INTEGUMENTARY ASSESSMENT" — Skin color within patient's norm. Skin clean, warm, dry and intact. Oral mucous membranes pink, moist and intact. No redness or lesions.

   g. "MUSCULOSKELETAL ASSESSMENT" — No joint swelling or tenderness. No pain, tenderness, or deformity in extremities. No pain or tenderness in back or neck. No ROM limitations. No muscle atrophy / weakness. Steady independent gait.

   h. "NEUROVASCULAR ASSESSMENT" — Affected extremity is warm and movable within patient's average ROM. CRT < 3 sec. Peripheral pulses palpable. No edema. Sensation intact without numbness or paresthesia.

   i. "SURGICAL DRESSING / INCISIONAL ASSESSMENT" — Dressing dry and intact. No evidence of redness, increased temperature, or tenderness in surrounding tissue. Sutures/ staples/ steri-strips intact. Wound edges well-approximated. No drainage present.

   j. "PAIN ASSESSMENT" — Patient is pain free or interventions were effective.

   k. "TUBE ASSESSMENT" — All Tubes are patent, no redness, drainage, or swelling at site of insertion. For Drainage tubes, no unexpected drainage is noted.

   l. "PSYCHO/SOCIAL ASSESSMENT" — Characteristics of appearance, behavior and verbalizations appropriate to situation. Alert and oriented to person, place and time. Memory intact. Affect appropriate. No mood swings noted.

   m. "CHEMOTHERAPY ASSESSMENT" — Chemotherapy delivered without adverse reaction. Patient in no acute distress. Labs checked prior to infusion. Good blood return established before, during and after delivery of every chemotherapy drug. No swelling or redness at IV site before, during, and after chemotherapy infused. IV site unremarkable after IV discontinued and until patient is discharged.

5. **NURSE INITIAL:** All entries must be initialed in the initial sections. RN must co-sign when appropriate.

6. **SIGNIFICANT FINDINGS:** Upon carrying out an order that has a significant finding, an asterisk is entered in the appropriate box. An asterisk * in this category box indicates to see integrated progress notes. Only abnormal or significant findings data (D) as well as any related actions (A) or response (R) are documented in the integrated notes.

7. **GENERAL INSTRUCTIONS:** If status remains unchanged from previous asterisk entry, current entry may be indicated with an "→".

8. **INITIATE FLOW:** When a new flow sheet is initiated, any abnormal data must be written out on the new flowsheet, whether previously described or not.

9. **DC ORDERS:** When orders are discontinued, enter D/C in next box.

10. **EQUIPMENT:** Enter type of equipment being used. When initiated, enter date and initials. When equipment is D/C, enter date and initials. When new form is initiated, then transcribe equipment still in use.

FIGURE 5.37 Continued.

Medical Center

ADMISSION PHYSICAL/RISK FOR FALLS ASSESSMENT

PHYSICAL ASSESSMENT PARAMETERS: The following parameters will be considered a normal assessment . If the physical assessment falls within the normal parameters listed below, indicate with a "✓" in the box following the specific assessment. A "＊" in the box denotes a finding that requires description on the lines to the right. Only exceptions to the norm will be documented on the lines or diagrams.

```
OS  1022      MR
              MO2,805   SCE
                1575
C5-10-37   60  F
```

Assessment Parameters	Exceptional Observations
NEUROLOGICAL ASSESSMENT — Alert and oriented to person, place and time. Behavior appropriate to situation. Pupils equal and reactive to light. No headache or visual disturbances. Active range of motion of all four extremities with symmetry of strength. No paresthesias or numbness. Verbalization clear and understandable. Memory intact. ✓	
CARDIOVASCULAR ASSESSMENT — Regular apical pulse. S_1, S_2 audible. Neck veins flat at 45 degrees. CRT less than 3 seconds. Peripheral pulses palpable. No edema. No calf tenderness. No chest discomfort. ✓	
RESPIRATORY ASSESSMENT — Respirations 12-20 per minute at rest. Respirations regular, quiet and easy without apparent effort. Breath sounds vesicular through both lung fields, bronchial over major airways. No adventitious sounds. Sputum clear. Nailbeds and mucous membranes pink. CRT < 3 seconds. ✓	
GASTROINTESTINAL ASSESSMENT — Abdomen flat, soft, pliant musculature when relaxed; Active bowel sounds all four quadrants (5-34 per minute). No ostomies. No visible or palpable masses. No pain with palpation. Tolerates diet without nausea or vomiting. Regular bowel pattern. ✓	
GENITOURINARY ASSESSMENT — Urine clear, yellow-amber in color. No palpable bladder distension. No catheter, ostomy. No dysuria or frequency. No urethral or vaginal discharge. ✓	
MUSCULOSKELETAL ASSESSMENT — No joint swelling or tenderness. No pain, tenderness or deformity in extremities. No pain or tenderness in neck or back. No limitations in range of motion. No muscle atrophy or weakness. Steady, independent gait. ＊	*Weakness in arms and leg. Has bilateral foot drop*

05100930＊

RN Signature _____   Date _10-22_   Time _0900_   ***Continue———***

FIGURE 5.38 Admission physical/risk for falls assessment.

ASSESSMENT PRAMETERS	EXCEPTIONAL OBSERVATIONS

INTEGUMENTARY ASSESSMENT
Skin color within patient's norm. Skin clean, warm, dry, and intact. No redness or lesions.
☑

IMPAIRED SKIN INTEGRITY - Assign a number to each area on the body diagram. Enter the number next to each characteristic that applies. You may have more than one number for each descriptor.

_____skin broken   _____red   _____draining

_____hot/inflamed   _____rashes   _____blisters

_____undermining   _____painful   _____induration

_____mottled   _____necrotic tissue (tan, yellow, black)

_____venous stasis changes   _____muscle/bone exposed

_____
_____
_____
_____

FOR PREDICTING PRESSURE SORE RISK - *BRADEN SCALE* - Complete for bed or chair bound patients and those who have Impaired ability to reposition.
Initiate appropriate Nursing Care Plan for total score ≤ 16.

Score

Sensory Perception
1. Completely Limited   2. Very Limited   3. Slightly Limited   4. No Impairment   _____

Moisture
1. Constantly Moist   2. Very Moist   3. Occasionally Moist   4. Rarely Moist   _____

Activity
1. Bedfast   2. Chairfast Occasionally   3. Walks Frequently   4. Walks   _____

Mobility
1. Completely Immobile   2. Very Limited   3. Slightly Limited   4. No Limitations   _____

Nutrition
1. Very poor   2. Probably Inadequate   3. Adequate   4. Excellent   _____

Friction & Shear
1. Problem   2. Potential Problem   3. No Apparent Problem   _____

(Score of 15-16 = low risk; 13 -14 = moderate risk; 12 or less = high risk)   **TOTAL** _____

PAIN ASSESSMENT
Patient is pain free
☑

PAIN CHARACTERISTICS AND INTENSITY
Assign a letter to each area of pain on the body diagram. Enter the letter next to each characteristic that applies. In the space provided, indicate pain scale used and patient's pain intensity.

_____Burning   _____Cramping   _____Sharp
_____Stabbing   _____Aching   _____Dull
_____Crushing   _____Deep   _____Radiating
_____Constant   _____Superficial   _____Localized
_____Intermittent   _____Throbbing   _____Incisional

_____
_____
_____
_____
_____

PAIN SCALE USED _numerical_
OVERALL PAIN RATING _O_

RISK ASSESSMENT TOOL (RAT) FOR FALLS

DIRECTIONS: Place a "✓" mark in front of elements that apply to your patient. The decision of whether or not a patient is at risk for falls is based on your nursing judgment.

GUIDELINE: A patient who has a "✓" mark in front of an element with an asterisk (*) or four or more of the other elements would be identified as at risk for falls.

General Data
☑ History of falls prior to admission*
☑ Postoperative/admit for operation
☑ Smoker   ☐ Age over 60

Ambulatory Devices Used
☐ Cane   ☐ Wheel chair
☐ Crutches   ☐ Geri chair
☐ Walker   ☐ Braces

Physical Condition
☐ Dizziness/Imbalance   ☐ Paresis
☐ Diarrhea   ☐ Unsteady gait
☐ Impairment of hearing   ☑ Weakness
☐ Impairment of vision   ☑ Urinary frequency
☐ Seizure disorder
☑ Diseases/problems affecting weight-bearing joints

Mental Status
☐ Confusion/disorientation*
☐ Impaired memory or judgment
☐ Inability to understand or follow directions

Medications
☐ Diuretics or diuretic effects
☐ Hypotensive or CNS suppressants (narcotic, sedative, psychotropic, hypnotic, tranquilizer, antihypertensive, antidepressant)
☐ Medication that increases GI motility (laxative, enema)

"Reprinted from Rehabilitation Nursing, 16(2), 167-169, with permission of the Association of Rehabilitation Nurses, 5700 Old Orchard Road, First Floor, Skokie, IL 60077-1057. Copyright © 1991 Association of Rehabilitation Nurses."

RN Signature_____   Date _10 -22-_   Time _0902_

FIGURE 5.38 Continued.

Medical Center

NURSING PROTOCOL

© AHC X9511 ID #413 (3/96)

DATE STARTED	INITIALS	DATE RESOLVED	INITIALS
10-34	AB		

FOCUS:
Post-op

PROTOCOL NAME:
Post-op Protocol: General Anesthesia

PATIENT / SIGNIFICANT OTHER INFORMED OF PLAN OF CARE ☒

Eval. Date	Initials
10-34	AB

EXPECTED OUTCOME(S):

Patient will obtain maximum level of wellness post-anesthesia and surgery as evidenced by:

a. Adequate airway and respiratory function

b. Adequate cardiac function and tissue perfusion

c. Adequate fluid and electrolyte balance and renal function

d. Adequate nutrition and elimination

e. No evidence of wound inflammation / infection

f. Return to pre-op mobility baseline

g. Verbalizing adequate pain relief and adequate sleep / rest pattern

DATE / INITIALS	FREQ.	PLAN:		DC Date / INITIALS
10-34 AB	As Listed	1. Initiate post-op protocol upon arrival to unit after surgery.		
	→	2. Post-op protocol to be continued on all patients for 24 hour after surgery. Post-op protocol may then be modified as needed at the discretion of the RN.		
	→	3. Minimum post-op vital signs: every 1° x 4, 10-34 AB every 4° x 24°, then every shift.		

IP 1024   MR
          M01,B05 SCE
05/10/37 60 F   1575

DATE / INITIALS	FREQ.	PLAN:		DC Date / Initials
10-34 AB	As Listed	4. Assessments to be implemented on all post-op patients at frequency of minimum vital signs and prn. a. Neurological assessment (level of consciousness and orientation) b. Cardiovascular assessment c. Respiratory assessment d. Surgical dressing / incision assessment e. Pain assessment / rating f. G.U. assessment g. G.I. assessment		
	→	5. Assessments to be implemented as needed: Frequency same as required assessments a. Neurovascular R U L b. Musculoskeletal c. Integumentary		
	→	6. Tube assessment per policy and procedure. Document at frequency of minimum vital signs and prn. Specify tubes: IV, JP drain		

FIGURE 5.39 Nursing care plan.

115

PROTOCOL INSTRUCTIONS

DATE STARTED: Enter date when began.
INITIALS: RN initiator initials

DATE RESOLVED: Enter date when protocol stopped.
INITIALS: Initials of RN discontinuing protocol.

FOCUS/PROTOCOL: Enter the focus word chosen to match the protocol title.

PATIENT/SIGNIFICANT OTHER: Check if patient/significant other involved in planning process. This must occur in a timely fashion after initiation of the protocol

EXPECTED OUTCOMES: Describe a goal in measurable terms.
EVAL. DATE/INITIALS: Determine a date to evaluate goal attainment. Enter RN initials. A progress note "R" entry should be done on eval. date.

PLAN: List activities necessary in the protocol.
FREQUENCY: List frequency in the FREQ. column.
DATE/INITIALS: Enter date of starting intervention and initials of RN planner.
DC DATE/INITIALS: Enter date when intervention stopped and RN initials.

DATE / INITIALS	FREQ.	PLAN:	DC Date / INITIALS

X9511

FIGURE 5.39 Continued.

116

Medical Center

TEACHING RECORD

```
DS 1022      MR
             M02,905  SCE
                 1575
C5-10-37  60 F
```

TEACHING CONTENT Module Title and Number	Objective	Patient	Sig. Other	First Time Teaching	Reinforcement	Verbalization Understanding	Return Demonstration
5/12	1	✓	✓	10·22	10·24 ✓	✓	
	2	✓		✓	✓	✓	
	3						
	4						
	1						
	2						
	3						
	4						
	1						
	2						
	3						
	4						
	1						
	2						
	3						
	4						
	1						
	2						
	3						
	4						
	1						
	2						
	3						
	4						
	1						
	2						
	3						
	4						
	1						
	2						
	3						
	4						

Significant Findings/Information:

05300260

TEACHING RECORD

FIGURE 5.40 Teaching record.

Medical Center

NURSING DISCHARGE
STATUS NOTE/INSTRUCTION SHEET

IP 1024   MR
M01.B05 SCE
05/10/37   60   F   1575

DISCHARGE:
Date 10-26-   Time 1445   Mode W/C

Accompanied by: FRIEND

DISPOSITION OF PATIENT:

☑ HOME   ☐ SPECIALTY CARE   ☐ NURSING HOME   ☐ OTHER _____

DATE: **TIME:**   Description of Patient Progress Toward Goal Attainment:

10/26/
1430

EXCELLENT RESSION TWDS. POST-OP
GWEN OUTCOMES OF PLAN OF CARE.
GOALS MET.

RN Signature _____

DISCHARGE PLAN AND INSTRUCTION SHEET

Discharge Medications or Prescriptions: ☑ Yes ☐ No   PERCOCET. PLS. REFER TO MED. INSTRUCTION SHEET.
Instructions given by: ☑ RN ☐ Pharmacist ☐ Other _____

Activity Limitations:

☐ Complete Rest   ☑ Frequent Rest Periods _____
☑ No Driving Car   UNTIL OK WITH DR.   ☑ Activity As Tolerated _____
☐ No Bending _____   ☑ Bathing SPONGE BATHS UNTIL OK WITH DR.
☑ No Heavy Lifting >15 LBS.   ☐ No Activity Limitations
☐ No Stair Climbing _____   ☐ May Resume Sexual Activity _____
☐ Other: (Describe) _____

Prescribed Diet: ☑ General   **Diet Instructions Given by:** ☐ Dietician ☐ Cardiac Rehab.
☐ Other _____   ☐ _____

Signs / Symptoms to watch for / Instructions:

– PLS. REFER TO YOUR FYWB AFTER GENERAL SURGERY AND CARE FOR YOUR
  JP DRAINS. CONTINUE TO DRAIN & RECORD YOUR DRAIN AS YOU'VE BEEN
  DOING EVERY 8 HRS. AND BRING THE RECORD TO YOUR MD'S VISIT.
– LEAVE SURGIBRA ON 24 HRS/DAY.

Appointments to be kept: APPT FOR TUE OR WED. WITH DR.   **Referral:** ☐ Yes ☑ No

Physician _____ Date _____   Agency: _____

I HAVE RECEIVED INSTRUCTIONS IN THE ABOVE AREAS AND UNDERSTAND THESE INSTRUCTIONS.

Patient Signature _____   Guardian Signature _____

RN Signature _____

05100940

NURSING DISCHARGE STATUS NOTE/INSTRUCTION SHEET

Printed on Recycled Paper

FIGURE 5.41 Nursing discharge status note/instruction sheet.

RESPIRATORY THERAPY PROGRESS NOTES
MEDICAL CENTER -

DIAGNOSIS _Right Breast CA_

OBJECTIVES _DB&C_

THERAPY _I.S._

IP 1024   MR

M01.B05 SCE

1575

DATE	TIME	MED		HR / RR	COUGH	SPUTUM		AUSCULTATION / COMMENTS
						COLOR	AMOUNT	15 / 10 / 3 7
								BS Clear I.S.
☐ HHN				a _58_ _18_	☐ NPC	☐ CLEAR	☐ SCANT	_instruct given 10_
☐ IPPB				P _79_ _16_	☐ WEAK	☐ WHITE	☐ SMALL	_breaths to 2500cc_
☐ USN	O2	☑ RM AIR	PEAK FLOW		☐ FAIR	☐ YELLOW	☐ MED	
☐ IPPB/USN	☐ N/C		a		☑ GOOD	☐ GREEN	☐ LARGE	
☐ CPT	MASK	☐ SIMPLE	P		☐ NONE	☐ BROWN	☐ COPIOUS	
☐ MDI	☐ NRBM	☐ TRACH			☐ SUCTION ORAL	☐ PINK	☐ THIN	
☐ IS	☐ AERO	☐ VENTURI	P/O ___ %		☐ SUCTION w/	☐ BLOODY	☐ THICK	
☐ TBT	LPM ___ % ___ Temp		Change s.u.		100% O2	☐ PALE	☐ FROTHY	
☐ VENT	CPAP	☐ NASAL		O2	SENSORIUM	☐	☐ MUCOID	
☐ ABG		☐ MASK			☐ RESPONSIVE			SIGNATURE
☐	CMH20 ___ %/LPM			Rx	☐ UNRESPON.			
TIME: 0930	☑ N/C ☐ MASK _2_ LPM _100_%	TIME 0930 P/O 95	HR 87 RA	SIGNATURE / DATE:
TIME:	☐ N/C ☐ MASK ___ LPM ___ %	TIME: P/O	HR	

DATE	TIME	MED		HR / RR	COUGH	SPUTUM		AUSCULTATION / COMMENTS
						COLOR	AMOUNT	
☐ HHN				a	☐ NPC	☐ CLEAR	☐ SCANT	_Found pt set_
☐ IPPB				P	☐ WEAK	☐ WHITE	☐ SMALL	
☐ USN	O2	☐ RM AIR	PEAK FLOW		☐ FAIR	☐ YELLOW	☐ MED	_up @ 24_
☐ IPPB/USN	☐ N/C		a		☐ GOOD	☐ GREEN	☐ LARGE	
☐ CPT	MASK	☐ SIMPLE	P		☐ NONE	☐ BROWN	☐ COPIOUS	_10/24_
☐ MDI	☐ NRBM	☐ TRACH			☐ SUCTION ORAL	☐ PINK	☐ THIN	
☐ IS	☐ AERO	☐ VENTURI	P/O ___ %		☐ SUCTION w/	☐ BLOODY	☐ THICK	_0930_
☐ TBT	LPM ___ % ___ Temp		Change s.u.		100% O2	☐ PALE	☐ FROTHY	
☐ VENT	CPAP	☐ NASAL		O2	SENSORIUM	☐	☐ MUCOID	_1025_
☐ ABG		☐ MASK			☐ RESPONSIVE			SIGNATURE:
☐	CMH20 ___ %/LPM			Rx	☐ UNRESPON.			
TIME:	☐ N/C ☐ MASK ___ LPM ___ %	TIME: P/O	HR	SIGNATURE / DATE:
TIME:	☐ N/C ☐ MASK ___ LPM ___ %	TIME: P/O	HR	

DATE	TIME	MED		HR / RR	COUGH	SPUTUM		AUSCULTATION / COMMENTS
						COLOR	AMOUNT	
☐ HHN				a	☐ NPC	☐ CLEAR	☐ SCANT	
☐ IPPB				P	☐ WEAK	☐ WHITE	☐ SMALL	
☐ USN	O2	☐ RM AIR	PEAK FLOW		☐ FAIR	☐ YELLOW	☐ MED	
☐ IPPB/USN	☐ N/C		a		☐ GOOD	☐ GREEN	☐ LARGE	
☐ CPT	MASK	☐ SIMPLE	P		☐ NONE	☐ BROWN	☐ COPIOUS	
☐ MDI	☐ NRBM	☐ TRACH			☐ SUCTION ORAL	☐ PINK	☐ THIN	
☐ IS	☐ AERO	☐ VENTURI	P/O ___ %		☐ SUCTION w/	☐ BLOODY	☐ THICK	
☐ TBT	LPM ___ % ___ Temp		Change s.u.		100% O2	☐ PALE	☐ FROTHY	
☐ VENT	CPAP	☐ NASAL		O2	SENSORIUM	☐	☐ MUCOID	
☐ ABG		☐ MASK			☐ RESPONSIVE			SIGNATURE:
☐	CMH20 ___ %/LPM			Rx	☐ UNRESPON.			
TIME:	☐ N/C ☐ MASK ___ LPM ___ %	TIME: P/O	HR	SIGNATURE / DATE:
TIME:	☐ N/C ☐ MASK ___ LPM ___ %	TIME: P/O	HR	

DATE	TIME	MED		HR / RR	COUGH	SPUTUM		AUSCULTATION / COMMENTS
						COLOR	AMOUNT	
☐ HHN				a	☐ NPC	☐ CLEAR	☐ SCANT	
☐ IPPB				P	☐ WEAK	☐ WHITE	☐ SMALL	
☐ USN	O2	☐ RM AIR	PEAK FLOW		☐ FAIR	☐ YELLOW	☐ MED	
☐ IPPB/USN	☐ N/C		a		☐ GOOD	☐ GREEN	☐ LARGE	
☐ CPT	MASK	☐ SIMPLE	P		☐ NONE	☐ BROWN	☐ COPIOUS	
☐ MDI	☐ NRBM	☐ TRACH			☐ SUCTION ORAL	☐ PINK	☐ THIN	
☐ IS	☐ AERO	☐ VENTURI	P/O ___ %		☐ SUCTION w/	☐ BLOODY	☐ THICK	
☐ TBT	LPM ___ % ___ Temp		Change s.u.		100% O2	☐ PALE	☐ FROTHY	
☐ VENT	CPAP	☐ NASAL		O2	SENSORIUM	☐	☐ MUCOID	
☐ ABG		☐ MASK			☐ RESPONSIVE			SIGNATURE:
☐	CMH20 ___ %/LPM			Rx	☐ UNRESPON.			
TIME:	☐ N/C ☐ MASK ___ LPM ___ %	TIME: P/O	HR	SIGNATURE / DATE:
TIME:	☐ N/C ☐ MASK ___ LPM ___ %	TIME: P/O	HR	

FIGURE 5.42 Respiratory therapy progress notes.

Medical Center

**Consent To Operation
or Other Procedures**

CS 1024.   MR
          M02,805 SCE
                    1575
CS/10/37   60   F

PATIENT NAME: _____

DATE: _____ 10·24- _____ TIME _____ 0815. _____ A.M.
                                                                            P.M.

1. (or_____ for_____) hereby
        (Name of person authorizing consent if other than patient)   (Name of patient)
   authorize Dr._____ and/or such assistants and designees
                (Name of physician who will perform the procedure)
   as may be selected by him/her, to perform a(n) *Right Segmental*
                                                   (Name(s) of procedures)
   Mastectomy and Right Axillary Lymph Node Dissection
   Right Modified Radical Mastectomy only if necessary.
   Also Node Mapping Procedure
   upon _____ *me* _____, if it is decided that it is advisable to
                ("Me" or name of patient)
   proceed with same.

2. I understand that the procedure is to be performed at   Medical Center, a
   teaching hospital. I hereby authorize Dr._____ to utilize, under
   his supervision, in the performance of the procedure, the services of other physicians,
   physicians who are receiving post-graduate medical training or medical students from the
   University of   Medical School or from the Medical College of

3. The procedure(s) to be performed have been explained to me by Dr._____
   _____ and I understand the nature of the procedure( ).

4. *(For Surgical Consents)* It has been explained to me that during the course of the operation, unforeseen conditions may be revealed that necessitate an extension of the
   procedure(s) or the performance of a procedure(s) other than or in addition to those set
   forth above. Therefore, I authorize and request that the above named physician, his
   assistants, or his designees perform such procedures as are necessary and/or desirable in the
   exercise of his (their) professional judgement.

5. I have been informed of the available alternative procedures and the possible complications, risks and consequences that are associated with the procedure(s) described above.

6. *(For Surgical Consents)* Further, I understand that there are other risks attendant to the
   performance of any surgical procedure. Such risks include, but may not be limited to, a
   severe loss of blood, infection, and cardiac arrest.

CONSENT TO OPERATION OR OTHER PROCEDURES

FIGURE 5.43 Surgical consent.

7. I have been informed that any previous DNR (Do No Resuscitate) order that may have been entered in my chart will be suspended during the procedure described above unless my chart includes documentation of agreement between me and my physician for the DNR order to continue throughout the procedure.

8. I am aware that the practice of medicine and surgery is not an exact science and I acknowledge that no guarantees have been made to me concerning the results of the operation(s) or procedure(s).

9. I hereby authorize _____ Medical Center, its agents, its employees and its designees, to examine, preserve for scientific or teaching purposes, or otherwise dispose of dismembered tissues, parts, or organs resulting from the procedure(s) authorized above.

10. I hereby authorize _____ Medical Center, its agents, its employees and its designees, to use as needed in living persons dismembered tissues, parts, or organs resulting from the procedure(s) authorized above.

11. I consent to the administration of anesthesia to be applied by or under the direction and supervision of a medical staff anesthesiologist, and to the use of such anesthetics as may be deemed advisable.

12. I consent to the photographing, filming, televising, or videotaping of the operation(s) or procedure(s) to be performed, including appropriate portions of my body, for medical, scientific, or educational purposes, provided my identity is not revealed by the pictures or by descriptive texts accompanying them.

13. I consent to the admittance of observers to the procedure room for the purpose of advancing medical education.

14. This Consent has been fully explained to me and certify that I understand its contents. All blanks or statements requiring insertion(s), completion or deletion were so adjusted before by signature was affixed below.

X _____   _____ *RN.*
Signature of Patient   Witness

15. The patient is unable to consent because:

  a. he / she is a minor _____ months / years of age.

  b. _____

  _____

  _____

_____   _____
Signature of Person Authorizing Consent   Witness

_____
Relationship to Patient

FIGURE 5.43 Continued.

_____ Medical Center

```
DS  ·'2-        ~:
                '·2,B_S  SC=
CS/·'C/3?  6?      F           :5.?
```

INPATIENT ADMISSION/OUTPATIENT
REGISTRATION AGREEMENT

GENERAL CONSENT TO CARE

I, the undersigned, for myself or a minor child or another person for whom I have authority to sign, hereby consent to medical care and treatment as ordered by my physician(s). This consent includes my consent for all hospital services, diagnostic procedures and medical treatment rendered under the general or specific instructions of a physician, including examinations, x-rays and laboratory procedures and other tests, treatments and medication, monitoring, blood transfusions, EKGs, and all the procedures, including invasive procedures, which do not require my specific informed consent. I understand that as a patient, I am under the direct care of physicians while in the Medical Center, and that the employees, agents and representatives of the Medical Center will carry out the instructions of those physicians. I further understand that almost all of the physicians who provide treatment to me while I am in the Medical Center are medical staff members and independent contractor physicians (including, but not limited to, emergency room physicians, anesthesiologists, radiologists, pathologists, and orthopaedic surgeons) who make decisions and take actions that are not under the control of the Medical Center. I agree and acknowledge that the Medical Center is not liable for the actions or omissions of, or the instructions given by such physicians who treat me while I am in the Medical Center.

PERSONAL VALUABLES

I understand and agree that the Medical Center assumes no liability for any loss of or damage to any money, jewelry, documents, furs, or other articles brought to the Medical Center. I understand the Medical Center security maintains a safe for the storage of money and valuables during inpatient hospitalization. I agree that the Medical Center assumes no control over personal valuables not deposited in its safe, and that no employee or agent of the Medical Center is authorized to suggest or recommend storage of such articles other than by security department personnel for inpatients in the Medical Center's safe.

RELEASE OF INFORMATION FOR BILLING PURPOSES

I hereby acknowledge and agree that the Medical Center and all physicians participating in my treatment may release to my insurers, other payors or other persons as necessary for billings and related purposes, at reasonable times and in accordance with the Medical Center policies and procedures, any information which may be needed for the purpose of billing, collection or payment of claims for services provided at or by the Medical Center. This information may include my identity, medical and psychological evaluations, diagnosis, prognosis and treatment for physical and/or emotional illness, developmental disabilities, treatment of alcohol or drug abuse, surgical procedures, progress notes, and all other information contained in patient care records, only to the extent that such

INPATIENT ADMISSION/OUTPATIENT REGISTRATION AGREEMENT

FIGURE 5.44 Conditions of Admission.

records are needed for billing or collection of benefits due me from any payor. I understand that I have a right, upon request, to inspect and receive a copy of all such records being disclosed. This authorization will terminate upon completion of all procedures and actions necessary for the billing, collection and payment of all claims related to services provided to me by the Medical Center for this inpatient stay or any Outpatient visits for one year.

RELEASE OF INFORMATION FOR DISCHARGE PLANNING

I hereby authorize the Medical Center and all physicians participating in my care to release to admission personnel representing home care agencies, nursing homes, subacute or other post-acute care facilities any information which may be needed to ensure my appropriate post-hospital placement.

ASSIGNMENT OF INSURANCE BENEFITS

I hereby authorize and assign payment directly to the Medical Center and its employed physicians, to Medical Center independent contractor and other provider based physicians of such hospital, and surgical expense insurance and other benefits and payments otherwise payable to me. I understand that I am financially responsible to the Medical Center for all amounts not paid by my insuror or other payor, provided that such charges are not in excess of the Medical Center's regular charges or a written contract between the Medical Center and a payor. I expressly promise and agree to pay the Medical Center, and any physician to whom I have assigned insurance benefits, all such charges which are not paid by either my insurance plan, PPO, HMO, or other coverage, in addition to copayments and deductible charges for services that are not covered by the Medicaid or Medicare programs. This Assignment is valid for one year.

_____	_____
Signature of Patient / Other	If other relationship
_____	_____
Date Signed	(Witness)

MEDICARE ASSIGNMENT AND ACKNOWLEDGEMENT

My signature below certifies that the information given by me in applying for payment under Title 18 of the Social Act is correct. I authorize any holder of medical or other information about me to release to the Social Security Administration or its intermediaries or carriers any information needed for services provided under this agreement or a related Medicare claim. I hereby request that payment of authorized benefits be made on my behalf to the Medical Center.

My signature below acknowledges my receipt, if I am an inpatient, of *"An Important Message From Medicare/ Champus"* from the Medical Center. However, my signature does not waive any of my rights to request a review of my care or make me liable for any payment except as described in "Assignment of Insurance Benefits."

_____	_____
Signature of Patient / Other	If other, relationship
_____	
Date Signed	

FIGURE 5.44 Continued.

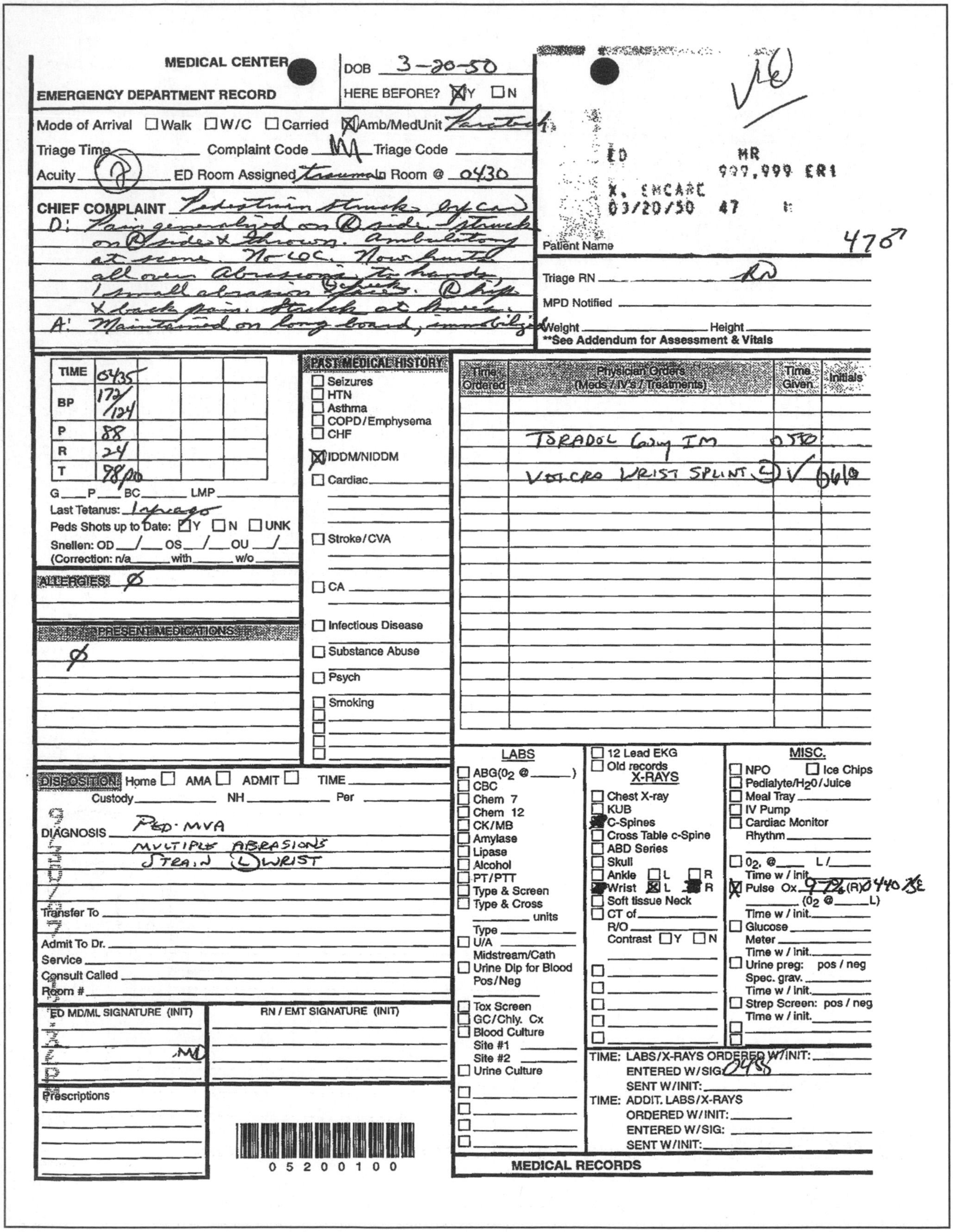

MEDICAL CENTER

EMERGENCY DEPARTMENT RECORD

DOB 3-20-50

HERE BEFORE? ☒Y ☐N

ED MR 999,999 ER1

X, EMCARE

03/20/50 47

Patient Name 47♂

Mode of Arrival ☐Walk ☐W/C ☐Carried ☒Amb/MedUnit Paratech

Triage Time ______ Complaint Code M Triage Code ______

Acuity (2) ED Room Assigned trauma In Room @ 0430

Triage RN RN

MPD Notified ______

Weight ______ Height ______

**See Addendum for Assessment & Vitals

CHIEF COMPLAINT Pedestrian struck by car

D: Pain generalized on (R) side. struck on (R) side & thrown. ambulatory at scene. No LOC. Now hurts all over. abrasions to hands, 1 small abrasion (R) cheek. (R) hip & back pain. Strick at knees.

A: Maintained on long board, immobilized

TIME	0435			
BP	172/124			
P	88			
R	24			
T	98 po			

G___P___BC___ LMP ___

Last Tetanus: 1yr ago

Peds Shots up to Date: ☐Y ☐N ☐UNK

Snellen: OD __/__ OS __/__ OU __/__

(Correction: n/a ___ with ___ w/o ___

ALLERGIES: Ø

PRESENT MEDICATIONS

Ø

PAST MEDICAL HISTORY

- ☐ Seizures
- ☐ HTN
- ☐ Asthma
- ☐ COPD/Emphysema
- ☐ CHF
- ☒ IDDM/NIDDM
- ☐ Cardiac
- ☐ Stroke/CVA
- ☐ CA
- ☐ Infectious Disease
- ☐ Substance Abuse
- ☐ Psych
- ☐ Smoking

Time Ordered	Physician Orders (Meds / IV's / Treatments)	Time Given	Initials
	TORADOL 60mg IM	0550	
	VELCRO WRIST SPLINT (L) ✓	0610	

DISPOSITION: Home ☐ AMA ☐ ADMIT ☐ TIME ______

Custody ______ NH ______ Per ______

DIAGNOSIS PED·MVA

MULTIPLE ABRASIONS

STRAIN (L) WRIST

Transfer To ______

Admit To Dr. ______

Service ______

Consult Called ______

Room # ______

ED MD/ML SIGNATURE (INIT) MD

RN / EMT SIGNATURE (INIT)

Prescriptions

05200100

LABS

- ☐ ABG(O2 @ ___)
- ☐ CBC
- ☐ Chem 7
- ☐ Chem 12
- ☐ CK/MB
- ☐ Amylase
- ☐ Lipase
- ☐ Alcohol
- ☐ PT/PTT
- ☐ Type & Screen
- ☐ Type & Cross ___ units
- Type ___
- ☐ U/A Midstream/Cath
- ☐ Urine Dip for Blood Pos/Neg
- ☐ Tox Screen
- ☐ GC/Chly. Cx
- ☐ Blood Culture Site #1 ___ Site #2 ___
- ☐ Urine Culture

☐ 12 Lead EKG

☐ Old records

X-RAYS

- ☐ Chest X-ray
- ☐ KUB
- ☒ C-Spines
- ☐ Cross Table c-Spine
- ☐ ABD Series
- ☐ Skull
- ☐ Ankle ☐L ☐R
- ☒ Wrist ☒L ☒R
- ☐ Soft tissue Neck
- ☐ CT of ___ R/O ___ Contrast ☐Y ☐N

MISC.

- ☐ NPO ☐ Ice Chips
- ☐ Pedialyte/H2O/Juice
- ☐ Meal Tray
- ☐ IV Pump
- ☐ Cardiac Monitor Rhythm ___
- ☐ O2 @ ___ L/ ___ Time w / init. ___
- ☒ Pulse Ox. 97% (R) 0440 KE ___ (O2 @ ___ L) Time w / init. ___
- ☐ Glucose Meter ___ Time w / init. ___
- ☐ Urine preg: pos / neg Spec. grav. ___ Time w / init. ___
- ☐ Strep Screen: pos / neg Time w / init. ___

TIME: LABS/X-RAYS ORDERED W/INIT: ______

ENTERED W/SIG: 0455

SENT W/INIT: ______

TIME: ADDIT. LABS/X-RAYS ORDERED W/INIT: ______

ENTERED W/SIG: ______

SENT W/INIT: ______

MEDICAL RECORDS

FIGURE 5.45 Portions of an emergency department record.

Medical Center

CBC		CHEMISTRY			ABG's	OTHER LAB RESULTS
Hgb	WBC	Na	Cl	BUN	ph	
Hct	Plt	K	HCO2	gluc	pCO2	
				Cr		
SEG		AMYLASE			pO2	
BAND		LIPASE			HCo3	
LYMPH		CK			O2 Sat	
MONO		MB			FiO2	
EO		ETOH				

ED   MR
                      999,999 ER1   9980
X,
03/20/50   47   M

Patient Name:

Case No.   :
Admitted   : 09/22/   0443
MRU   :
Physicians : X,

TIME SEEN _____

47 year old black male.
Patient was involved in a(n) accident approximately 1 hour prior to arrival. The patient was a pedestrian.
Struck by auto at low speed. Patient complains of neck and left wrist pain with several scattered abrasions.
There has been no apparent head trauma. There are no other complaints.

REVIEW OF SYSTEMS: as above.
PMH: diabetes
SOCIAL HISTORY: noncontributory.
PHYSICAL EXAM: Vital Signs: Reviewed Nurse's notes.
PATIENT STATUS: alert and cooperative.
HEAD: No sinus tenderness.
Mild tenderness of the right cheek with superficial abrasion . No scalp tenderness.
EYES: PERRL, EOMI without nystagmus, no discharge or injection.
NECK: The patient arrived immobilized.
Cervical spine was cleared by X-ray. No cervical spine tenderness. Mild paravertebral tenderness. Range of
motion: full.
CHEST: No tenderness.
LUNGS: Clear to auscultation and breath sounds equal, no wheezes, rales, or rhonchi.
HEART: Regular rate and rhythm without murmurs, ectopy, gallops, or rubs.
BACK: No costovertebral, paravertebral, intervertebral, or vertebral tenderness or spasm.
PELVIS: Nontender and stable to palpation.
ABDOMEN: Soft, nontender, without masses.
NEUROLOGICAL: Alert and cooperative. Sensory and motor functions intact.
GAIT: normal.
EXTREMITY: Left wrist Tender, nonswollen, Range of motion: full. No deformity. Skin is abraded. Also with
superficial abrasions to bilateral hands, knees and right thigh. Normal distal neurovascular status
X-RAY: left wrist and C-spine-no acute changes
INTERVENTION:
Velcro wrist splint was applied to the left wrist.
Toradol 60mg IM was given. After treatment the patient's pain was mostly relieved.
DIAGNOSIS:
Abrasion: Multiple Sites, 919.0
Sprain: Left Wrist, 842.00
Patient was a pedestrian that was hit by a motor vehicle. E814.7

DISPOSITION: Patient was discharged home. The patient's condition at discharge was satisfactory.
The following prescriptions were given to the patient: ibuprofen 800mg po q6-8 hours prn #20.
See the chart for further detailed instructions given to the patient and/or family.
Instruction sheets for abrasion and contusion and sprain were given.
The patient was advised to follow-up with the patient's personal physician in 1-2 days.
Patient/family instructed to return to the ED if symptoms worsen prior to PMD follow-up.

                        M.D.
              Mon Sep 22, 19 , 06:50 AM

CONDITIONS ON DISCHARGE: ☐ IMPROVED ☐ UNCHANGED

                                               SIGNATURE   M.D.

05206896   **EMERGENCY PHYSICIAN TREATMENT RECORD**
0 5 2 0 6 8 9 6   05206896

FIGURE 5.45 Continued.

RECORD OF DEATH

ADDRESSOGRAPH

Date _____

1. Name in Full _____

   Address _____

2. Age _____ Sex _____ Color _____ Room _____

3. Date of Admission _____ 19 _____ Hour _____

4. Date of Death _____ 19 _____ Hour _____

5. Service of Dr. _____

   Address _____ Phone No. _____

6. Apparent Cause of Death _____

7. Nurse Present _____ Supervisor Notified By _____

8. Pronounced Dead By _____ Time _____

   Remarks _____

9. Next of Kin _____ Notified _____

   Address _____ Phone No. _____

10. Attending Physician Notified By _____ Time _____

11. Is Post Mortem Requested? _____

12. Did Operation Precede Death? _____ If Yes, Type of Operation _____

13. Coroner Name _____ Case No. _____

FUNERAL DIRECTOR RECEIPT

RECEIVED FROM ~~PLACENTIA LINDA~~ COMMUNITY HOSPITAL

The Body Of _____

Order Given By _____

Body Released By _____ Date _____ Time _____
                    SIGNATURE

List Valuables _____

_____

Body Received By _____ Valuables Received B, _____
                    SIGNATURE   SIGNATURE

Funeral Home _____ Phone No. _____

FIGURE 5.46 Record of death.

Memorial Hospital

TRANSFER FORM

HMH Admit Date: _____ Diagnosis:_____

*Transferring MD:_____*Accepting MD: _____

*Facility Accepting Transfer:_____Date:_____Time:_____

Report Given To:_____by Whom: _____

*Reason for Transfer: ☐ Specialized equipment not available at HMH.

        ☐ Specialized services not available at HMH.

        ☐ Other_____

*Patient Status: ☐ Critical   ☐ Stable   Code Status: No / Full / Chem Only

Advanced Directive: ☐ No ☐ Yes _____

Transfer Mode / Unit: ☐ Flight   ☐ Ambulance — Name: _____

        ☐ Police   ☐ Other_____

Sent with Patient:

☐ Medical Records/face sheet   ☐ Progress Notes   ☐ X-ray Report/Films
☐ H & P   ☐ M.D. Consults   ☐ EKG/Telemetry
☐ Discharge Summary   ☐ Lab Results   ☐ Maternal Blood
☐ NSG Data Base   ☐ Med Sheet   ☐ Cord Blood
☐ Pt. Belongings (List & Location)_____

*RISK OF TRANSFER

☐ Possible deterioration of condition   ☐ Accident in route
☐ Increased pain   ☐ Harm to fetus if pregnant
☐ Increased bleeding   ☐ No improvement of condition
☐ Possible loss of limb   ☐ Possible complication
☐ Possible infection   ☐ Other _____

PATIENT INFORMATION AT TIME OF TRANSFER

Allergies: _____

Time:_____   BP: _____

    T_____   P_____   R_____

Pulse Ox:_____O2: _____

Telemetry: ☐ No ☐ Yes

Rhythm: _____

IV's: _____

_____

Foley:_____NG: _____

Other: _____

_____

SYSTEMS ASSESSMENT:

☑ = WNL   ☐ = Abnormal

☐ Neuro _____
☐ Pulmonary _____
☐ CV _____
☐ GI _____
☐ GU _____
☐ Peripheral Vasc _____
☐ Integumentary _____
☐ Psychosocial / Emotional _____
☐ _____

*AUTHORIZATION FOR DISCLOSURE:

☐ I have been informed of the risks and benefits of transfer and acknowledge there are no guarantees related to the outcome of this transfer, (if applicable)

☐ I also authorize disclosure of information from my health care records pertinent to my current medical condition

☐ I do not want HIV test results to be disclosed

Date _____   _____
        SIGNATURE OF PATIENT

Date _____   _____
        SIGNATURE OF PERSON AUTHORIZED BY PATIENT

Authorization for disclosure will remain in effect for ninety days.   MD Signature_____

* Starred items do not need to be completed for in-house transfer.   RN Signature: _____

TRANSFER FORM   ORIGINAL -   / COPY - ACCEPTING FACILITY

FIGURE 5.47 Transfer record.

ANTEPARTUM SUMMARY

GR	P	AB	AGE	EDC	WK GEST	Time last food	Allergies	Breast ☑YES ☐NO	Rh & Type	Membranes Ruptured	DATE	TIME
2	1	0	26	12/10	40	AM	Epidural		A Neg	FLUID ☑ Clear ☐ MEC TR +1+2+3	12/8	1700

COMPLICATIONS OF PRIOR OR CURRENT PREGNANCY	PEDIATRICIAN	FETAL MONITOR		
Denies		☑External 75.34 ☐Internal Electrode 75.32	Onset of Labor	12/8 1700

| DR. | TIME NOTIFIED 1440 | TYPE OF LABOR ☑Spontaneous ☐Induced Augmented | ☐Internal Pressure Catheter | Admit to Hospital 12/8 1441 Complete Cervical DIL 12/8 1620 |

Antepartum Maternal Data
- ☐ Hypertension — 642.2
- ☐ Infection Type _____
- ☐ Seizure Disorder — 780.3
- ☐ Diabetes (class _____) — 648.0
- ☐ Anemia — 648.2
- ☐ Pregnancy Induced Hypertension — 642.3
- ☐ Eclampsia — 642.6
- ☐ Medications (list)

- ☐ Substance Abuse (specify drug) — 648.3

- ☐ Weight over 200 lbs. — 646.1
- ☐ Fetal Demise (currently) — 656.4
- ☐ Other (specify) _____

Previous Pregnancy Complications
- ☐ Premature Delivery — V23.4
- ☐ Previous Stillborn — V23.5
- ☐ Previous C/S (state indication) — 654.2

Present Complications
- ☐ No Prenatal Care
- ☐ Premature Labor — 644.0
- ☐ PROM — 658.1
- ☐ Prolonged ROM + 12 hrs. — 658.2
- ☐ Incompetent Cervix — 654.5
- ☐ Third Trimester Bleeding — 641.9
- ☐ Mutiple Gestation (twin) — 651.0
- ☐ Over 42 weeks — 645.0
- ☐ Abnormal Presentation(transverse lie)652.3
  - Breech _____ — 652.–
- ☐ IUGR — 656.5
- ☐ Placental previa — 641.1
- ☐ Placenta abruptio — 641.2

Special Procedures
- ☐ Amniocentesis — 75.1
- ☐ Prostaglandin — 96.49
- ☐ Ultrasound
- ☐ Tocolysis

Labor Complications
- ☐ Abnormal Bleeding — 641.9
- ☐ Maternal Fever — 659.2
- ☐ Foul Smelling Fluid — 658.4
- ☐ Meconium Fluid — 656.3
- ☐ PIH — 642.3
- ☐ Prolonged Labor — 662.1
- ☐ Prolonged 2nd Stage — 662.2
- ☐ Tachycardia — 656.3
- ☐ Bradycardia — 656.3
- ☑ Variable deceleration — 656.3
- ☐ Prolonged deceleration — 656.3
- ☐ Late deceleration — 656.3
- ☐ Minimal variability — 656.3
- ☐ Tetanic contractions — 661.4
- ☐ Prolapsed Cord — 663.0
- ☐ Failure of dilation — 661.–
- ☐ Arrested labor — 661.–
- ☐ Other _____

DELIVERY SUMMARY

DATE OF BIRTH 12-8-XX	TIME 1717	SEX GIRL	WEIGHT GMS 2890	LBS. 6	OZ. 6	LENGTH 19 4Pcm	BIRTH ☑LIVE ☐ STILLBORN ☐ NEONATAL DEATH

APGAR 1 MINUTE TOTAL: 8	5 MINUTE TOTAL: 9	ID BAND NO. 2536	APPLIED IN DR. BY R~	MECONUM IN DR. ☑ NO ☐ YES	SUCTION ☑OROPHARYNX ☐ TRACHEA

Placenta Expulsion at: 17.35	No. of Vessels: 3	☐Nuchal cord x _____	MEDICATION IN DELIVERY 10 Kitocin to IV fe placent	DOSE	TIME	SIGNATURE

☑Spontaneous
☐ Manual 75.4
☐ Abruption 641.2

☑ Cord blood ☑to lab
Cultures Yes ☐ Reason _____
No ☑

Presentation	Vertex	C/S		Laceration	
☑ vtx OA	☑Spontaneous	☐ Primary	☐ Herpes 647.6	☐ None	
☐ vtx OP	☐ Fundal Pressure	☐ Repeat 654.2	☐ Other _____	☐ 4th Degree 664.3	
☐ Breech	☐ Low forceps 72.1	☐ Classical 74.0	**Episiotomy**	☐ 3rd Degree 665.2	
☐ Other _____	☐ Vacuum ext. 72.71	☐ Transverse 74.1	☑None	☐ 2nd Degree 665.1	
Stages	☐ BOA	**Indication for C/S**	☐ Midline _____ 73.6	☑1st Degree 664.0	
First _____	**Breech**	☐ CPD 653.4	☐ Mediolateral 73.6	**Anesthesia**	
Second _____	☐ Spontaneous 72.52	☐ Fetal Distress 656.3	☐ Extension	☐ Local	
Third _____	☐ Assisted 72.51	☐ Abnormal	☐ EBL >500 cc 666.1	☑Epidural	
	☐ Forceps 72.51	Presentation 652.3		☐ Spinal	
				☐ General	

Complications Noted in Delivery Room Ø		Support Person Present in DR. (Yes) No

DELIVERED BY:	ASSISTING Ø	PED. PRESENT AT DELIVERY Ø

ANESTHESIOLOGIST Dr	DELIVERY ROOM NURSE RN	NEWBORN CARE NURSE

CIRCULATING NURSE RN	COMMENTS	

SCRUB NURSE RN		

OBSTERICIAL NURSING SUMMARY

FIGURE 5.48 Delivery record.

HOSPITAL NEWBORN RECORD SHEET

NAME	OBSTETRICIAN	PEDIATRICIAN
Tse		

Mother: Age 38 Gr 2 P 1 Ab ___ EDC 12-14-XX Type/Rh O+ Serology NR Rubella Imm Hepatitis Positive
Complications Previous Pregnancies: Ø
Complications This Pregnancy: mother + for Hep. B
Labor Onset: Date 12-17-XX Time 2300 (Spont.)/Induced Membrances Ruptured: Date 12-18-XX Time ___
Amniotic Fluid: (Normal)/Meconium ___ /Odor ___ Fetal Distress: Yes/(No)
Medications given to mother: (Type, date, time) ___ Anesthesia: Yes/(No) - Type ___
Delivery: (Spont.)/Forceps/C-Sect-Indication ___ Comment: ___
Placenta: (Normal)/Abnormal ___ Cord: (Normal)/Abnormal ___

		Apgar	1MIN	5MIN		Comments:
Birthdate	12-18-XX				Suction: (Bulb)/(Wall)/DeLee	
Birth time	0917	HR	2	2	Oxygen: Blow-by for ___ min	
Weight (g)	3365	Reflex	2	2	Bag & Mask for ___ min	
(lbs)	7-6	Resp	2	2	Intubation for ___ min	
Length (in)	21"	Tone	2	2	Cords Visualized: Yes / No	
Head (cm)	34 cm	Color	0	1	Cords Clear: Yes / No	
Boy/(Girl)	(Breast) (Y)/N	Totals	8	9	Other:	
Baby Blood Type		Signature:			M.D./(R.N.)	

Physical Exam	Normal	Comments
General	✓	
Color	✓	
Head	✓	
Eyes	✓	
Ears	✓	
Nose/Throat	✓	
Clavicles/Thorax	✓	
Respiratory	✓	

Comments:

Physical Exam	Normal	Comments
Cardiac	✓	
Abdomen	✓	
Hips	✓	
Genito-urinary	✓	
Skin	✓	
Moro/Grasp	✓	
Suck	✓	
Tone	✓	

Impression: Gest. Age 40 week (Newborn) Male/(Female) (AGA)/LGA/SGA
Signature: ___ M.D. Date 12-18-XX Time 1000

PROGRESS NOTES: (Please date & time)

12-18-XX Admit note —
Healthy ♀ via NSVD ̄s prob.
Px WNL no prob ̄c HbSAg ⊕ mom
will give HBIG + VACCINE

12/19/XX Day 1. Wt. 3340 g
Doing fine on breast
O/E normal color
Chest clear
CVS — no murmur
S1S2 normal
abdo — soft, no masses
Hips normal
Imp healthy infant
Home today
Plan Continue series of Hepatitis vaccine.

DISCHARGE DIAGNOSIS:
(Newborn) M/(F) (Term)/Preemie/Post
(AGA)/LGA/SGA
Other Dx: ___

Followup: 1 week in office

Signature: ___ *M.D.*

MR 0000
BABYGIRL
F 000H

WHITE-Chart Copy YELLOW:Nursery Copy PINK: Physician Copy

FIGURE 5.49 Newborn physical record and progress notes.

SUMMARY

Each document found in a medical record is designed to streamline the documentation process and, at the same time, meet statutory and regulatory agency requirements. Their correct placement into the record ensures that retrieval of information necessary for continuation of patient care and other uses is not impaired.

LEARNING ACTIVITIES

1. Discuss the purpose of the discharge summary, operative report, history and physical, and consultation report.

2. Explain how laboratory results are to be filed.

3. What is the purpose for having a specific chart order?

4. Discuss the components that may be found in specialty records, such as obstetrical, newborn, rehabilitation, and psychiatric records.

5. What are the advantages to using permanent record dividers?

6. Match the form with the correct purpose of the documentation.

Form	Purpose of Documentation
___ (a) History and physical	(1) Consent to basic treatment/agree to pay for services
___ (b) Consent	(2) Specialist's exam and findings
___ (c) Progress notes	(3) Patient understands need for procedure, risks, benefits; agrees to proceed
___ (d) Consultation report	(4) Mother's medical history, progress notes through pregnancy
___ (e) Prenatal records	(5) Synopsis of patient's treatment during an episode of care
___ (f) Medication administration record	(6) Demographic and insurance information
___ (g) Conditions of admission	(7) Focus of care and expected outcomes
___ (h) Discharge summary	(8) Daily report of patient diagnosis, treatment, and so on
___ (i) Face sheet	(9) Past medical treatment and current examination of body
___ (j) Delivery record	(10) Time and amount of medications given to patient
___ (k) Nursing care plans	(11) Specifics of fetal delivery and Apgar rating at 1 and 5 minutes

## CHAPTER 6

Analysis of the Record

ADT system	A computer system that records hospital admissions, discharges, and transfers.
Attending physician	The physician responsible for the total care of the patient throughout hospitalization.
NCR	A form that makes duplicates without carbon paper.
Physician privileges	Those services that a physician is permitted by the medical staff to perform in a healthcare facility. Examples of privileges are admitting a patient, consulting, and performing surgery.
Suspension	Temporary restriction of a physician's privileges as a penalty for having delinquent medical records.

OBJECTIVES

When you have completed this chapter you will be able to:

- Discuss the reason for analysis of the record after discharge.
- Determine who has responsibility for completing each portion of the record.
- Review a record and identify omissions of required documentation.

COMPLETION REQUIREMENTS

As we discussed in Chapter 2, the medical record provides continuity of care for the patient and serves as a legal document. In order to meet these requirements, the record must have documentation that is as complete as possible. This means that all test results are in the record, that all reports have been dictated, and that all documentation is authenticated by the persons making entries. It is the health information management department's responsibility to ensure that the record is complete once the patient has been discharged. Consequently, all HIM departments have written procedures for conducting analysis of the record after discharge. The completion requirements are based on state and federal law, Joint Commission on the Accreditation of Healthcare Organizations (JCAHO) standards, and the individual hospital medical staff bylaws, rules, and regulations.

Time Frames

JCAHO standards allow thirty days from the date of patient discharge for the record to be completed, unless the state law has a more stringent requirement. California, for example, allows only fourteen days for the record to be completed. Medical staff bylaws, rules, and regulations usually allow temporary **suspension** of **physician** admitting, clinical, and surgical **privileges** when a physician has delinquent records for a specified number of days. In order to give the physician ample time to complete the record and avoid suspension, the HIM department must perform **analysis** on an ongoing and efficient basis. This usually means that the record is analyzed within two to three days after discharge.

ANALYSIS

Once the record is assembled, the analysis clerk goes through the record page by page and looks for omissions in documentation or missing signatures. Each page must contain the patient's name, medical record number, and a date on which that particular documentation was made. Later if the record is taken apart, or documents are accidentally torn out, their proper replacement is ensured. This check also ensures that documents belonging to a different patient are not filed in the wrong record.

HISTORY AND PHYSICAL

The admitting physician writes or dictates the history and physical report (H&P) within 24 hours of patient admission to the hospital. The H&P can be done up to seven days prior to admission. If the patient is being admitted for surgery, the physical exam must be updated no more than 24 hours prior to the procedure and the H&P must be in the record prior to the start of the procedure. These are JCAHO requirements.

To check that the H&P was dictated within 24 hours of admission, check the last page of the report. The date and time dictated are recorded. Compare it with the date and time of admission recorded on the facesheet. To check that the H&P was in the record before surgery, check the Operating Room Nurse's record for the date and start time of the surgery and compare them with the date and time the H&P was dictated.

Physicians who do not meet the time requirements may be reported to the appropriate medical staff committee.

Interim H&P

If the patient is readmitted within thirty days, the physician does not need to prepare an entire H&P. He or she needs only to update the physical exam and state any changes in the patient's condition or that no changes have occurred. This is known as an interim H&P.

Short H&P

Most outpatient procedures also require an H&P. However, some hospitals allow physicians to use a short H&P format. The short H&P may contain a checkoff portion for the basic physical examination. The physician then adds the reason for the procedure. For example, a patient with carcinoma who becomes anemic may be admitted as an outpatient for a blood transfusion. The physical condition of the patient that is pertinent to the blood transfusion is the laboratory result of the hemoglobin and hematocrit. Other physical aspects are probably not that pertinent to the need for the transfusion. In this case, a short H&P is all that is needed. Note that requirements for H&Ps on outpatient procedures will vary by hospital.

CONSULTATION REPORTS

When analyzing a record, check the physician orders to see what consultations were ordered. Then, check to make sure you have a report for each consultation ordered. If there is not a separate report, check the progress notes because the consultant may have written the report on a progress note form. As we discussed in Chapter 5, consultation reports should document that the consultant has reviewed the medical record and has examined the patient.

A surgical consultation may be written or dictated by the surgeon prior to surgery so that the report will be on the record before the patient actually goes to the operating room.

Operative Reports

Operative or procedure reports should be written or dictated immediately after surgery. As with the H&P, check the date of the report against the actual date of the surgery. An operative report must include the surgeon's and assistant surgeon's names, pre- and postoperative diagnoses, the procedure(s) performed, findings, and a description of the procedure. The description includes the estimated blood loss, any blood or fluids given to the patient, drains and tubes placed, and the patient's condition at the conclusion of the procedure.

The surgeon is required to write a postoperative progress note immediately after surgery. The note must include the names of the surgeon and any assistants, the pre- and postoperative diagnoses, the procedure performed, findings, and specimens removed. In order to ensure that the physicians complete this type of progress note, some hospitals use a rubber stamp (Figure 6.1), or a preprinted progress note form, that lists the required information directly in the progress note. All the physician has to do is to fill it in and sign it.

DISCHARGE SUMMARY

Ideally, the discharge summary should be written or dictated at the time of patient discharge from the hospital, while the events of the patient's hospitalization are clear in the attending physician's mind.

Determining Attending Physician

Part of the analysis procedure is determining who should dictate the discharge summary. It should be the **attending physician,** but determining which physician is the attending physician is not always easy. For example, the patient may be admitted by Dr. Adams, who is in a group with Drs. Bond and Currin. The patient is actually a regular patient of Dr. Bond, but he is on vacation. Dr. Adams treats the patient for the majority of the hospitalization, but Dr. Bond comes back from vacation a few days before the discharge and actually writes the discharge order. If the discharge summary is assigned to Dr. Adams, he may do it or he may say that the patient is really Dr. Bond's patient and Dr. Bond should dictate the discharge summary.

Another problem can occur with discharge summaries when a surgeon is involved. The patient may be admitted by a family practitioner, Dr. Dolan, who calls in a surgical consultant, Dr. Elgin. Dr. Elgin takes over the case, performs the surgery, and writes the discharge orders. It is natural to assume that Dr. Elgin is going to do the discharge summary. However, she may decide that because she was the sur-

```
┌─────────────────────────────────────────────────────┐
│  DATE:        PRE-OP DX:                             │
│  POST OPERATIVE DX:                                 │
│                                                     │
│  PROCEDURE:                                         │
│                                                     │
│                                                     │
│  SURGEON:                                           │
│  ASSISTANT:                                         │
│  ANESTHESIA:                                        │
│  EST. BLD. LOSS:                                    │
│  BLOOD & FLUIDS:                                    │
│  DRAINS & TUBES:                                    │
│  POST-OP COND:                                      │
│  SIGNATURE:                                         │
└─────────────────────────────────────────────────────┘
```

FIGURE 6.1 Rubber-stamped surgical note used if there will be a delay in transcription of the operative report.

geon and Dr. Dolan was actually the attending physician following the patient, Dr. Dolan should dictate the discharge summary.

Determining who the attending physician is will depend on the individual physicians in your hospital, your medical staff rules and regulations, and health information management department policies and procedures.

TEST RESULTS

Test results, such as EKGs and x-rays, that require interpretation must be authenticated by the physician making the interpretation. Pathology reports require the authentication of the pathologist. When conducting analysis, you may be asked to determine that a test report exists for every test ordered. This can be accomplished by checking the orders to see which tests were requested. Then check the progress notes to determine which tests were actually performed and the date. Use this information to check against the reports that have been filed. As with any portion of the record that you find missing, always check the documents that have not yet been filed before marking the omission as a deficiency.

*O*RDERS AND PROGRESS NOTES

All orders must be signed by the physician giving the order. Be particularly careful to check verbal and telephone orders in which the doctor's name is written down by the nurse taking the order. Usually, an order must be signed by the physician within 24 to 48 hours of the order being taken by the nurse. Check to ensure that a physician has written a discharge order.

Some hospitals require that progress notes be checked to ensure that they are signed. In addition, you may check to see that an admitting progress note has been written by the admitting physician. Even if the patient stays only one day, there must be some documentation of the treatment given. It is possible that you will find only an admission note and a discharge note.

*A*NESTHESIA RECORDS

The JCAHO requires that the anesthesiologist write a preanesthesia note as well as a postanesthesia note. Both notes must be dated. The postanesthesia note must also be timed because the JCAHO requires that the note be written within 24 hours following discharge from the recovery room.

*N*URSING AND ANCILLARY SERVICES RECORDS

Most HIM departments do not conduct analysis of nursing and ancillary department records because these departments should be conducting their own quality reviews. However, there are still HIM departments that do analyze for nursing deficiencies and documentation. Items that may be checked include the admission database signed by an RN and the discharge status note that documents the date and time of discharge, the patient's condition at discharge, and to where the patient was discharged. Medication administration records are checked to ensure that an RN has signed for all shifts, even if no medication is given.

*D*EFICIENCY SLIPS

In order to conduct analysis of the record, there must be a system to show where the omissions in documentation are located in the record and to differentiate between the different physicians who must complete the record. A **deficiency slip** (Figure 6.2) is used for this purpose. Usually a separate slip is filled out for each physician who must make an entry in the record.

Colored Indicator Strips

In order to differentiate between the different physicians, the health information management department will use some sort of colored indicator (Figure 6.3). These are usually small strips of colored plastic that have adhesive on one side. Each physician is assigned a color, and the strips are placed at the edge of the page near the item to be completed (Figure 6.4). The colored indicator is also placed on the deficiency slip pertaining to that particular physician.

When the physician comes into the HIM department to complete records, he or she need only look at the deficiency slip to determine the color used to mark his or her deficiencies. The physician then looks for all of the tags of that color.

MR # _____

CHART DEFICIENCY SLIP

	DICTATE/COMPLETE	SIGN
Face Sheet	_____	_____
Discharge Summary	_____	_____
Condition on Disch.	_____	_____
Final Diagnosis	_____	_____
History & Physical	_____	_____
Consultation	_____	_____
Progress Notes	_____	_____
Pre-op Prog. Note	_____	_____
Post-op Prog. Note	_____	_____
Operative Report	_____	_____
Physician Orders	_____	_____

Other:_____

_____

_____

_____

PATIENT NAME _____ DISCH. DATE _____

PHYSICIAN _____

FIGURE 6.2 An example of a manual deficiency slip.

Preprinted Deficiency Slip

The deficiency slip is normally preprinted with the items to be checked when conducting analysis. When you find an omission in documentation, indicate on the deficiency slip that the physician must either complete a report (for example, dictate a discharge summary) or sign a report or order. Also indicate on the deficiency slip the patient's name, discharge date, analysis date, and the physician's name.

Computerized Deficiency Slip

In a computerized system, enter into the computer the patient's medical record number, discharge date, name, analysis date, physicians' names, and the particular deficiencies. If there is an interface with the admission, discharge, transfer (**ADT**)

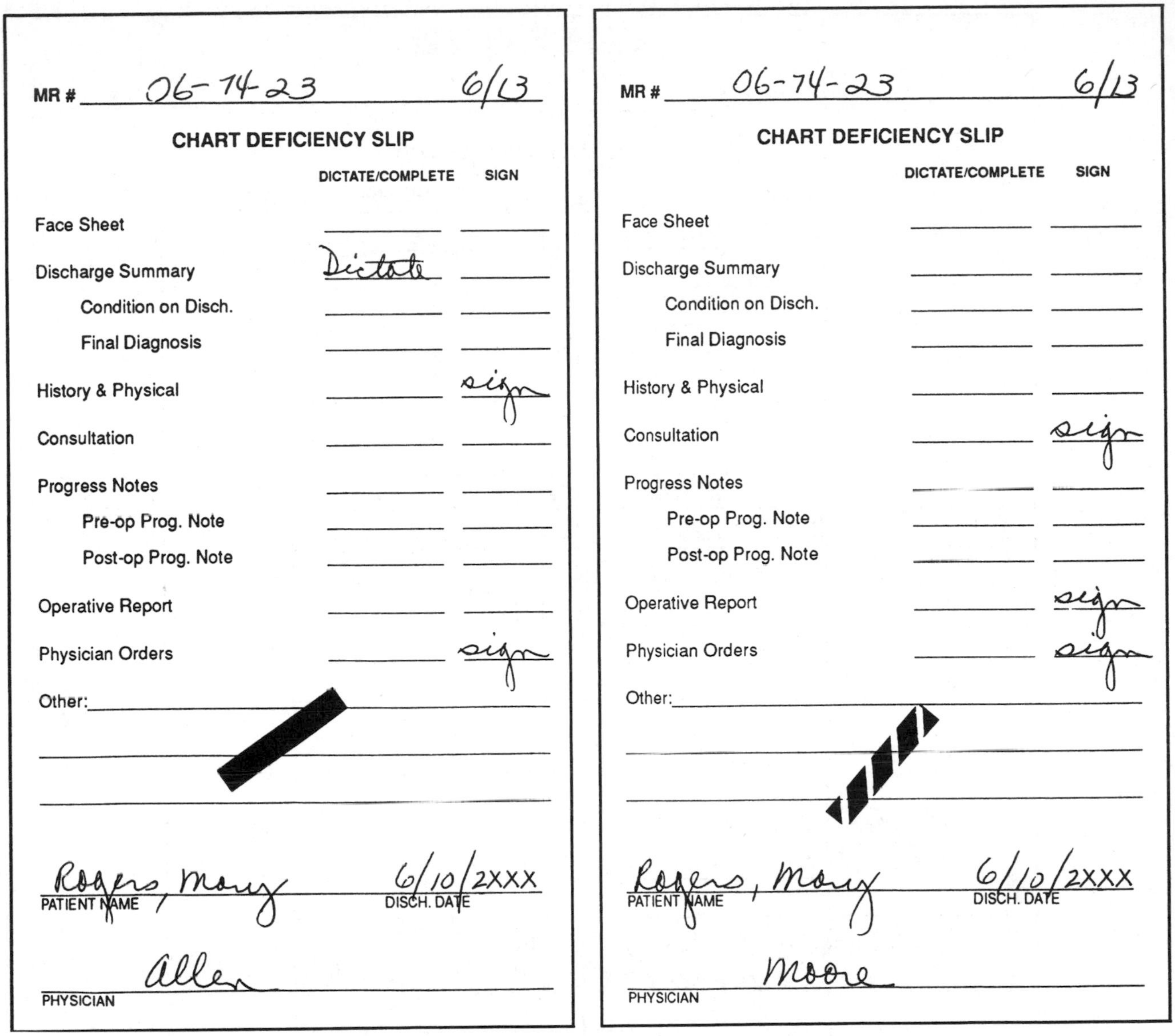

FIGURE 6.3 Deficiency slips for two physicians on a single record.

system, the patient information and treatment dates will be automatically placed in the deficiency system. Once all the deficiencies have been entered, the computer (Figure 6.5) will print out a deficiency sheet listing all physicians and deficiencies for that record. The computer may also be instructed to print a separate deficiency slip for each physician with the items to be completed.

Use of Slips to Pull Records

The manual deficiency slip is usually an original with one **NCR** copy. The original slip goes into the medical record and the copy is then filed by physician name. When a physician visits the department to complete records, all of the deficiency slips for the physician are pulled and used to retrieve the records. In a health information management department using a computerized system, a list of the physician's incomplete records is printed out at the time the physician visits the department. This eliminates the need for keeping deficiency slip copies. Different methods for ensuring that the physician completes all records will be discussed in Chapter 7.

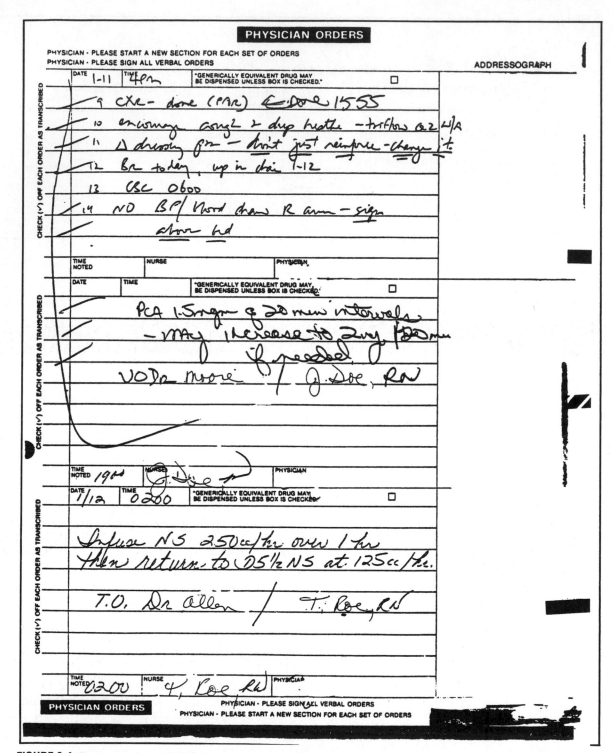

FIGURE 6.4 Documentation with deficiency tags corresponding to the deficiency slips in Figure 6.3.

```
                        CHART DEFICIENCY SHEET


     RECORD # 06-68-88    DISCH DATE: 07/04/2XXX   PATIENT: BYRD/MATTHEW
--------------------------------------------------------------------------
       DOCTOR            LVL    DEFICIENCIES·                   COLOR
--------------------------------------------------------------------------

      MARTIN/EDWARD       dict   DISCHARGE SUMMARY


      EWING/JAMES         dict   OPERATIVE REPORT


      HERRERA/DANIEL             SIGNATURES ONLY
```

FIGURE 6.5 Computerized deficiency slip.

SUMMARY

The medical record serves both as a legal document and as documentation of patient treatment to be used for effective continuation of treatment. In order to serve these functions, the documents in the record must be as complete as possible. The HIM department must check to ensure that all reports are completed and that all entries are authenticated.

LEARNING ACTIVITIES

1. What is meant by the phrase "conducting analysis of the medical record"?

2. Why is analysis conducted and what is its importance?

3. Fill in the blanks.
   (a) The JCAHO requires that all records be completed within _____ days after discharge.
   (b) The postanesthesia note must be written by the anesthesiologist within _____ hours after administration of the anesthetic.
   (c) The H&P must be completed within _____ hours after admission.
   (d) Telephone/verbal orders must be signed by the physician within _____ hours of giving the order.
   (e) If a patient is readmitted within _____ days, an interim H&P may be written rather than preparing a new H&P.
   (f) The operative report must be completed _____ after surgery.

4. Listed in Column A below are components of the medical record. In Column B are documentation requirements. Match the requirements in Column B to the components listed in Column A. Use as many in Column B for each item in Column A as necessary.

Column A	Column B
Discharge summary	Date
H&P	Patient name
Test results	Time
Consultation report	Medical record number
Operative report	Dictated
Anesthesia record	Written
Progress notes	
Physician orders	
Admit note	
Discharge order	

5. Explain the difference between manual and computer-generated deficiency slips and why the slips are used.

6. You have analyzed the record of patient Robert Mason, discharged on February 21, 2XXX. Create deficiency slips to annotate the following deficiencies. Write the tag colors on the slips if tags are not available. Do not discard the slips. They will be used in the Chapter 7 exercises.

Dr. S. Jones—Dictate discharge summary
    Sign H&P
    Sign orders
    Sign progress note

Dr. D. Martin—Sign consultation report
    Dictate procedure note
    Sign orders

Dr. T. Jones—Dictate consultation report
    Sign EKG report
    Sign orders

Dr. N. Owens—Sign orders
    Time postanesthesia note

Physician Incomplete Area

Complete record   A record containing all required documentation and authentications.

Delinquent record   A record that remains incomplete longer than the time allowed by medical staff bylaws, rules, and regulations.

Doctor's box   A method of filing incomplete records by physician rather than by medical record number.

Incomplete record   A record containing deficiencies in documentation.

JCAHO accreditation   Three-year approval given when a hospital meets the standards for providing quality healthcare.

Suspension list   A list of all physicians whose privileges are currently restricted because of delinquent medical records.

When you have completed this chapter, you will be able to:

- State the completion time frames required by the JCAHO as well as the acceptable delinquent record level.

- State the sequence of notification letters to physicians, the purpose of each, and the result.

- Demonstrate an understanding of the proper and positive way to communicate with physicians.

- State the difference between an incomplete and delinquent record.

- Demonstrate the procedure for retrieving a physician's records, assisting with completion, and checking the records after they are completed.

Working in the physician incomplete area can be one of the more interesting jobs that a medical record clerk can perform; it can also be one of the most stressful.

COMPLETION REQUIREMENTS

Complete Record

The JCAHO requires that all records of inpatients be completed within thirty days of discharge. This means that all entries are authenticated, all reports are completed, and all documents that should be in the record are present.

State Regulations

Some states also have regulations regarding the completion time for a medical record after discharge. For example, in California, a record must be complete within fourteen days of discharge. Other states, such as Wisconsin, Oklahoma, Texas, and Florida, have no state-mandated time frames for completion. These states rely on the JCAHO standard of thirty days after discharge. Your hospital's procedure for incomplete/delinquent records will be based on the JCAHO's standards as well as any state law.

Medical Staff Rules

The medical staff at each hospital will determine its own rules for record completion and these will be stated in the medical staff bylaws, rules, and regulations. For example, a hospital may use a standard of fourteen days that the record is considered to be incomplete. After fourteen days the record is considered **delinquent.** At twenty one days the physician may be suspended if he or she has not completed the records.

$\mathscr{P}$HYSICIAN NOTIFICATION PROCEDURE

The department procedure for notifying physicians about incomplete/delinquent records might be as follows, in a state with a fourteen-day completion requirement. When the physician has incomplete records seven days postdischarge, the health information management department sends a reminder letter stating that the records will be delinquent in one week. This letter is usually sent as a courtesy and may not be required by the medical staff bylaws, rules, and regulations. At fourteen days postdischarge, a delinquent letter is sent. This letter may state that the physician has records that are considered delinquent, and if they are not completed within one week, the physician's admitting, clinical, and surgical privileges will be temporarily suspended until the records are completed.

This notification process seems like a simple procedure, but in actuality it can have many difficulties. For example, not all physicians have records delinquent at the same time, so the health information management department must decide at what point to send the letter; otherwise, it would have to send delinquent letters every day. Most departments are not staffed sufficiently to allow daily letters. Therefore, the department usually picks a date and on that date checks all physician lists of records to be completed.

First Letter

If a particular physician has records that have been added only within the last seven days, the first letter (Figure 7.1) is sent. In addition, the first letter may be sent if the physician has a delinquent record that was not available when he or she came into the department. Most departments do not hold a physician responsible for a record that was not available.

Delinquent Letter

If the physician has records that are incomplete fourteen days postdischarge, the delinquent letter (Figure 7.2) is sent.

MERCY MEDICAL CENTER
4445 E. Short Street
Anywhere, CA 99999

June 5, 2XXX

John Doe, M.D.
555 S. Apple Street
Anywhere, CA 99999

Dear Doctor:

Since your last visit, additional medical records have been analyzed and added to your computer list. A copy of the list is enclosed. Please visit the HIM department soon to complete them. They will not be considered delinquent until June 12, 2XXX.

During the last JCAHO survey, the hospital received a Type I recommendation because of delinquent medical records. The next progress report is due to the JCAHO in August. In order to maintain accreditation we must reduce the number of delinquent records. Please do your part in reaching the goal.

If you have any questions or feel that the computer list contains errors, please contact Janet Mallory, Director, HIM at 999-9999.

Sincerely yours,

James Samuels, M.D.
Chief of Staff

FIGURE 7.1 Incomplete record notification letter.

Suspension Letter

If the physician has records that are twenty-one days old and he or she has been sent the delinquent record letter, the physician's office is called and reminded that the physician will be suspended the following day if the records are not completed. If, on the following day, the physician fails to come to the department and complete the records, a suspension letter (Figure 7.3) is sent to him or her by certified mail. This letter states that the privileges are being temporarily suspended because of delinquent records and requests that the physician contact the health information management department as soon as possible to arrange for completion.

Suspension List

Once he or she is suspended, the physician's name is placed on the **suspension list,** which is routed throughout the hospital. A physician who is suspended is not allowed to admit patients, perform consultations on any patient, or perform any procedures. A surgeon will not be allowed to operate on any patient. The suspended physician is, however, expected to continue care for any inpatients being treated at the time suspension was enforced. Patient care cannot be compromised for any reason.

MERCY MEDICAL CENTER
4445 E. Short Street
Anywhere, CA 99999

June 5, 2XXX

John Doe, M.D.
555 S. Apple Street
Anywhere, CA 99999

Dear Doctor:

Enclosed is a list of your incomplete medical records. Any record with a discharge
date prior to May 20 is considered delinquent. These must be completed by June
12 to avoid suspension.

During the last JCAHO survey, the hospital received a Type I recommendation
because of delinquent medical records. The next progress report is due to the JCAHO
in August. In order to maintain accreditation we must reduce the number
of delinquent records. Please do your part in reaching the goal.

If you have any questions or feel that the computer list contains errors, please
contact Janet Mallory, Director, HIM at 999-9999.

Sincerely yours,

James Samuels, M.D.
Chief of Staff

FIGURE 7.2 Delinquent record notification letter.

JCAHO Accreditation

We have previously discussed reasons for having a complete and legible medical
record; another reason involves JCAHO surveys of the hospital. If the number of
delinquent records is too high, the hospital may lose its accreditation. When a hospital loses its **JCAHO accreditation,** it may not treat Medicare patients, a primary
source of income.

$\mathcal{N}$OTIFICATION PROCEDURE FOR ONE PHYSICIAN

Let's take a look at the notification procedure for a particular physician over a one-
month period (Figure 7.4). On February 1, Dr. Jones's list of records is examined. He
has no records that are past the fourteen-day postdischarge status. Therefore, he is
sent a first courtesy letter. On February 8, one week later, Dr. Jones's list is checked
again. He now has records that are incomplete fourteen days postdischarge, and he is
sent a delinquent letter. On February 15 the list is checked again. Dr. Jones has one
record that is outstanding twenty one days postdischarge, but all the other records
that were delinquent the previous week have been completed. Upon checking, the

MERCY MEDICAL CENTER
4445 E. Short Street
Anywhere, CA 99999

June 5, 2XXX

John Doe, M.D.
555 S. Apple Street
Anywhere, CA 99999

Dear Doctor:

In accordance with our medical staff bylaws, your medical staff privileges have been suspended as of June 12, 2XXX, because of delinquent medical records.

This suspension includes all admitting, consultative, and operative procedures.

Physicians who have accumulated 30 or more suspension days in any twelve-month period may be reported to the Medical Board.

Please contact Janet Mallory, Director, HIM at 999-9999 to arrange for completion of your records as soon as possible.

Sincerely yours,

James Samuels, M.D.
Chief of Staff

FIGURE 7.3 Suspension letter.

Date	Status of Records After Discharge	Letter Sent
2/1	No records greater than 14 days	1st courtesy letter
2/8	Greater than/equal to 14 days	Delinquent letter
2/15	All complete except one record over 21 days that is unavailable	1st courtesy letter
2/22	Greater than/equal to 14 days	Delinquent letter
3/1	Greater than/equal to 21 days	Suspension letter

FIGURE 7.4 Chronological status of one physician's records and resulting correspondence.

medical record clerk finds out that the record was not available; it could not be located. Because it was not Dr. Jones's fault that the record was not completed, he is again sent a first courtesy letter, because all of his records are now less than seven days postdischarge or were unavailable for completion.

On February 22 the list is checked again. Dr. Jones has not been in. The records now are incomplete fourteen days postdischarge, so he is sent a delinquent letter. On March 1, the list is checked again. Dr. Jones still has not completed his records; they have been available. Dr. Jones's office is called; he is told that he is about to be suspended and that he has until 2 P.M. the following afternoon to complete the records. On March 2, Dr. Jones comes in and completes all the delinquent records that require signature but he does not do the dictations. In this case, Dr. Jones must still be suspended because all delinquent records must be completed to avoid suspension. Therefore, a suspension letter is sent by certified mail to Dr. Jones.

SUSPENSION LETTER SIGNATURE

Suspension notification letters may be signed by the health information management director, the chief of staff, or the hospital administrator. This will vary depending on the needs and desires of the particular hospital and medical staff.

PROCESSING SUSPENSION LIST

The list of suspended physicians (Figure 7.5) is sent to all hospital departments that deal with physicians, such as admitting, emergency room, operating room, and the nursing units. It is the responsibility of these departments to enforce the suspension

---

Date: July 10, 2XXX

To: All Departments

From: Sue Dawson, RHIA
        Director, HIM

Subj: Physician Suspension

The following physicians have been suspended because of delinquent medical records. Until further notice, they may not admit, perform consultations or procedures, or perform surgery.

James Allen, M.D.

Roxanne Beaudette, M.D.

Richard Jones, M.D.

George Chambers, M.D.

Horton Byrd, M.D.

FIGURE 7.5 Suspension list routed to all departments.

policy. It is the HIM department's responsibility to ensure that the list is always current. As soon as a physician has completed his or her records, he or she must be removed from the list, and a new list must be circulated to all of the departments so that they do not deny privileges to a physician who actually is off the list. Many computerized chart tracking/deficiency systems contain an option to count suspension days, by physician, to facilitate reporting.

*I*NCOMPLETE RECORD FILING

Doctor's Box

There are two methods by which incomplete records can be filed while they are awaiting completion by the physicians. The first is called the **"doctor's box"** method. All of the records for a particular physician are placed behind that physician's name and remain there until he or she has completed them. For example, the record of Amy Chen needs to be completed by Drs. Allen, Beaudette, and Chambers. The record is placed in Dr. Allen's box. Once he has completed it, it is placed in Dr. Beaudette's box, and once Dr. Beaudette has completed it, it is placed in Dr. Chambers's box. In a hospital with a low census and a small medical staff, this system can work. However, in any other type of hospital, the doctor's box system is not very efficient. If the record is placed in Dr. Allen's box and Dr. Beaudette comes in to complete her records before Dr. Allen, the record of Amy Chen will not be available for Dr. Beaudette to sign. If Dr. Allen is notoriously behind in completing his records, the chart of Amy Chen may not be completed for four or five months. Hospitals that use the doctor's box system usually have a master list for each record stating which physicians must complete the record. In that way they are able to check each doctor's box for the record and pull it out if Dr. Beaudette comes in before Dr. Allen. Again, however, this method requires much cross-checking and can often be in error.

Terminal Digit

A more efficient method, and the one used by most hospitals, is to file the records in terminal digit order. Any record can be pulled, at any time, for any reason, and the location of the record, for the most part, is always known. Some hospitals file **incomplete records** in strict terminal digit order. Others file by only the last two digits. This is because the records are pulled in and out of the file so often that the amount of time spent putting the records in strict terminal digit order is greater than the time to search the particular terminal digit for the correct record.

*P*ULLING RECORDS FOR PHYSICIAN COMPLETION

As a medical record clerk in the physician incomplete area, you will be required to pull records for physicians when they want to complete them. Some physicians will call or stop by ahead of time to let the department know when they will arrive. Others just show up. The majority of physicians are very busy and do not like to wait. Physicians often come into the department to complete their records when they have a few minutes between conducting morning rounds and morning office hours or between lunch and afternoon office hours.

$\mathcal{S}$ TEP-BY-STEP PROCEDURE FOR PULLING RECORDS

When pulling records for physician completion, you must work quickly using a procedure such as the following.

1. **Pull Deficiency Slips**
   Go to the physician's file and pull out all of the **deficiency slips** for his or her records; or, if the department has a computer system, print out a list of the records.

2. **Place Slips in Terminal Digit Order**
   If there is time, put the deficiency slips in strict terminal digit order or by the last two digits, depending on the filing system.

3. **Pull the Records**
   Start pulling the records. If the hospital files each episode of care separately until it is complete, compare the discharge date on the deficiency slip with the discharge date on the chart. You must make sure that you have the correct episode of care, because the patient may have more than one. If the wrong episode is pulled, the physician is likely to sign another physician's entry or may fail to complete his or her own record. If the physician is waiting, pull two or three records and give them to him or her so that he or she can start working while the rest of the records are pulled.

4. **Pull Easily Found Records First**
   If a record cannot be found, put that slip aside. Pull the records that can be easily found first, then start searching for the others. If using a computer system, pull up that particular record on the screen and see which other physicians need to complete it. It is possible that one of the other physicians has called ahead and asked that his or her records be pulled. The record needed for Dr. Allen may be in Dr. Beaudette's stack. If Dr. Chambers has been in on the previous day and dictated a report, the record may be in a separate area waiting for the transcribed report to return from transcription. Or, the patient may have been readmitted since he or she was last discharged, and the record has been delivered to the nursing station. The record may have been pulled for correspondence or for audit purposes or any number of reasons.

5. **Search Records Pulled for Other Physicians**
   If a computer system is not available to identify which other doctors have requested the record, start searching through those records that have been pulled for other physicians. The fastest way to look for a record is, again, by using the color-coded terminal digits. Look for the colors rather than the actual number.

6. **Document Record Not Found**
   If, after searching diligently, a record still cannot be located, cross through the analysis date on the deficiency slip and write the current date. This documents that the physician came by to complete the record but the record was not available. If using a computer system, there may be a way to enter this information into the computer.

7. **Ask Physician Intentions**
   If all of the records cannot be found when a physician is waiting, ask him or her if he or she will be coming back later. If not, there is no point in trying to find the records that are currently unavailable. They probably will be available next time. However, if the physician is willing to wait or if he or

she has a large number of records that have already been pulled, it is important for you to know where to look in the health information management department and other departments for those records that need completion. Ideally, all records requiring completion should be pulled every time the physician visits the department.

*P*HYSICIAN INCOMPLETE AREA

When all records are pulled for a physician who has called ahead, place them in the **physician incomplete area** with a note on top that contains the doctor's name and the date the records were pulled. The fact that a physician calls ahead to have his or her records pulled does not mean that he or she will come to the department. The physician may get busy in the office and not have the time or may simply forget.

Time Limit

Most departments have a time limit as to the number of days that the records may sit in the incomplete area before being refiled. This may be from 48 hours up to one week. The reason for having such a rule is to maintain efficiency in the department. The more records that are pulled out under doctors' names, the more difficult it is to find records when physicians actually do come in to complete them. If the physician does not complete the records before the department time limit is exceeded, refile the deficiency slips in the physician's file and refile the records in the incomplete file.

*W*ORKING WITH PHYSICIANS

Some physicians often do not like "paperwork"; completing medical records is considered paperwork. Therefore, visiting the health information management department to complete medical records is usually a low priority for them. For a few, a visit to the HIM department to complete records occurs only when they are threatened with suspension or are actually suspended.

Stressed Physicians

While working in the physician incomplete area, you may meet physicians who exhibit signs of stress. This usually happens when the physician is overworked, worried about a patient, or has just had a bad day. Such behavior should not be taken personally, because it usually is not directed personally.

Incentives

Many HIM departments provide positive reinforcements such as candy and other "goodies" as rewards for the physicians who do their records. Others conduct contests among the physicians to see who does his or her records in the most timely manner, with the winner receiving some kind of gift. When you have worked in the incomplete area for a time, you will learn the different physician personalities and how to handle them. There are, however, some basic ideas to remember about working with physicians.

Know the Record

You must know the record itself, backward and forward. If a physician asks why he or she is being asked to complete a document or write a note, you must be able to explain why. Although the physicians should know what the record completion requirements are, some do not. Therefore, it is your job to be able to explain the requirements. Physicians also may not be familiar with the order of the medical record forms. A physician may ask for help in finding a particular laboratory report. It is necessary to know the chart order as well as the documentation requirements.

Communication

When conversing with a physician, speak clearly and distinctly. Be courteous. Remember, every employee has the responsibility for good customer service. If a physician thinks hospital staff are discourteous or are not offering the services required, he or she may take patients elsewhere. You are not required, however, to accept verbal abuse. If a problem arises, let your supervisor handle the situation. It is wise to report any such problem to your supervisor so that a physician complaint later can be followed up. Remember, you should not talk back to a physician or exhibit anger. It is not easy to keep cool under some of the situations that occur in the health information management department, but the reality is that you will need to be prepared to deal in a calm, informed, courteous, and mature fashion with a variety of physician personalities.

Know the Medical Staff

In order to deal effectively with a physician, you need to know what his or her specialty is, who his or her partners are, and what kind of dictation or records he or she normally completes. This will alert you to potential errors in analysis. For example, a consultant, such as a pulmonary specialist, may infrequently dictate discharge summaries. A family practitioner is unlikely to dictate an operative report.

$\mathcal{R}$ EPORTING PROBLEMS

If you are able to successfully solve a physician complaint, the actual complaint and how it was resolved should be reported to your supervisor, because the complaint itself may indicate a problem in some other area of the HIM department. For example, if a physician states that he or she dictated a discharge summary but the transcribed report cannot be found, this may indicate a problem with the hospital dictation system. The supervisor needs to know about this so he or she may check it out and make sure that there is no problem or that the problem is corrected.

$\mathcal{U}$ PDATING FILES AFTER COMPLETION

Once the physician has completed the records, go through each record to make sure that each item listed on the deficiency slip has been completed. If an item is complete, pull the indicator tag off of the record. Some hospitals reuse the indicator tags. Others place the tag on the deficiency slip in the area pertaining to the item that was completed. For example, if a progress note was marked for signature, remove the indicator tag from the progress note and place it over the check mark (Figure 7.6) under "sign progress note" on the deficiency slip. This procedure is used as another check before deleting the item from a computerized system.

Missed Item

If a physician completed all items but missed one signature on a record, circle that item on the deficiency slip and make some note. When the physician looks at that deficiency slip the next time, he or she will ensure that the particular item is com-

MR #	06-93-35	6/17

CHART DEFICIENCY SLIP

	DICTATE/COMPLETE	SIGN
Face Sheet	_____	_____
Discharge Summary	_____	_____
Condition on Disch.	_____	_____
Final Diagnosis	_____	_____
History & Physical	_____	_____
Consultation	_____	_____
Progress Notes	_____	✓
Pre-op Prog. Note	_____	_____
Post-op Prog. Note	_____	_____
Operative Report	_____	_____
Physician Orders	_____	_____
Other:_____		

Martinez, Joe   6/15/2XXX
PATIENT NAME   **DISCH. DATE**

Wong
PHYSICIAN

047-010036 (6/90)

MR #	06-93-35	6/17

CHART DEFICIENCY SLIP

	DICTATE/COMPLETE	SIGN
Face Sheet	_____	_____
Discharge Summary	_____	_____
Condition on Disch.	_____	_____
Final Diagnosis	_____	_____
History & Physical	_____	_____
Consultation	_____	_____
Progress Notes	_____	_____
Pre-op Prog. Note	_____	_____
Post-op Prog. Note	_____	_____
Operative Report	_____	_____
Physician Orders	_____	_____
Other:_____		

Martinez, Joe   6/15/2XXX
PATIENT NAME   **DISCH. DATE**

Wong
PHYSICIAN

047-010036 (6/90)

FIGURE 7.6 Deficiency slip before and after the physician's visit to the incomplete area. All items have been completed.

pleted. Also check to make sure that the indicator tag is sticking out from the page far enough so that the physician can identify where it is. If the tag is placed too far inside the page, the physician may miss it.

Dictated Report Pending Transcription

If the physician has dictated a report, such as a discharge summary, the record must be refiled pending transcription of the report. Some hospitals mark the date the report was dictated on the front of the file folder in pencil, and file the record in a separate area. Others simply refile the record in the incomplete area. Once the transcribed report has been received, the deficiency slip and record must be updated. File the report in the record in the correct area, and place the correct color of indicator tag where the signature should be. Cross out "dictate" on the deficiency slip and write in "sign" (Figure 7.7). Then refile the deficiency slip and the record.

MR # _06-14-23_   6/17

CHART DEFICIENCY SLIP

	DICTATE/COMPLETE	SIGN
Face Sheet	_____	_____
Discharge Summary	*Dictate*	_____
Condition on Disch.	_____	_____
Final Diagnosis	_____	_____
History & Physical	_____	*sign*
Consultation	_____	_____
Progress Notes	_____	*sign*
Pre-op Prog. Note	_____	_____
Post-op Prog. Note	_____	_____
Operative Report	_____	_____
Physician Orders	_____	*sign*
Other:	_____	

Garcia, Maria   6/15/2XXX
PATIENT NAME   DISCH. DATE

Chambers
PHYSICIAN

MR # _06-14-23_   6/17

CHART DEFICIENCY SLIP

	DICTATE/COMPLETE	SIGN
Face Sheet	_____	_____
Discharge Summary		*sign*
Condition on Disch.	_____	_____
Final Diagnosis	_____	_____
History & Physical	_____	_____
Consultation	_____	_____
Progress Notes	_____	_____
Pre-op Prog. Note	_____	_____
Post-op Prog. Note	_____	_____
Operative Report	_____	_____
Physician Orders	_____	_____
Other:	_____	

Garcia, Maria   6/15/2XXX
PATIENT NAME   DISCH. DATE

Chambers
PHYSICIAN

FIGURE 7.7 Deficiency slip prior to physician dictation and updated after report is received from transcription.

Transferring Completion to Another Physician

If a physician requests that a record be given to another physician for dictation of a report, honor that request. On the deficiency slip put "Dr. Allen, per Dr. Chambers." This lets Dr. Allen know that it was Dr. Chambers who requested that he do the discharge summary and not the HIM department. If Dr. Allen then says that it is not his record and that Dr. Chambers should dictate the summary, give it back to Dr. Chambers, "per Dr. Allen." If Dr. Chambers then still refuses to dictate the summary, refer the problem to the supervisor for resolution. Do not let physicians play "table tennis" with the record more than once before reporting the problem to your supervisor.

COMPUTERIZED DEFICIENCY SLIP

Hospitals with computerized systems have the option of printing out a new deficiency slip (Figure 7.8) each time a change is made or simply making the change in the computer and updating manually the deficiency slip itself. It is extremely important that the computer system be updated daily so that the statistics on the number of incomplete/delinquent records are accurate and so that the physician lists are accurate. It is very embarrassing for a department director to suspend a physician for delinquent records when that physician has actually completed the records and the computer system has not been updated.

FINAL CHECK

Once all physicians have completed a particular record, that record may then go to final check. Final check is a last check before the records are filed permanently to ensure that all documentation is complete. It is usually a quick check of only major items. For example, check to ensure that there is a dictated and signed H&P and discharge summary and that all progress notes and orders are signed. If the patient has had surgery, the hospital may check for a dictated and signed operative report and pre- and postanesthesia notes from the anesthesiologist. Some hospitals then mark the record with a "C," or some other mark on the face sheet, to indicate that the record is **complete.** The record is then filed in the permanent file area. Final check is not routinely performed in most hospitals because of time and staffing constraints.

RECORD FILED INCOMPLETE

A record may not be filed incomplete in the permanent file unless the medical staff instructs the health information management director to do so. This usually only happens in a case where a physician has moved out of the area or has died without completing all of his or her records.

```
                        CHART DEFICIENCY SHEET

   RECORD # 06-68-88    DISCH DATE: 07/04/2XXX   PATIENT: BYRD/MATTHEW
   ----------------------------------------------------------------------
     DOCTOR                LVL   DEFICIENCIES               COLOR
   ----------------------------------------------------------------------

    MARTIN/EDWARD         dict   DISCHARGE SUMMARY


    EWING/JAMES           sign   OPERATIVE REPORT


    HERRERA/DANIEL               SIGNATURES ONLY
```

FIGURE 7.8 Computerized deficiency slip before physician completion and after Dr. Ewing has dictated operative report.

DELINQUENT RECORD STATISTICS

The JCAHO requires that delinquent record statistics be reported to the medical staff by the HIM department. A medical record clerk working in the physician incomplete area may be asked to provide the statistics or help generate them. A computerized system is usually programmed to provide the number of incomplete and delinquent records. It can also provide the number of records that have a specific deficiency (e.g., H&P not dictated).

Number of Delinquent Records Acceptable

If a hospital is to retain its JCAHO accreditation, the number of delinquent records may not exceed one-half of the average monthly discharges for the hospital. For example, if the hospital discharges an average of 500 patients per month, the number of delinquent records may not exceed 250. The definition of a delinquent record is based on the hospital medical staff bylaws, rules, and regulations.

At the time of JCAHO survey, the health information management director completes a form that shows the average number of delinquent records for each of the four quarters before the survey. The four quarterly numbers are averaged and the total compared with the average monthly discharges for the previous twelve months. If the number of delinquent records is greater than 50 percent of the discharges, the hospital will receive a Type I recommendation. A percentage of 100 or more results in conditional accreditation, which requires the hospital to develop a corrective action plan, submit periodic progress reports, and possibly be resurveyed. If the number of delinquent records is 200 percent or greater, the surveyors will recommend loss of accreditation for the hospital.

The quarterly number is derived by averaging the number of delinquent records for each of the months of the quarter. The count of delinquent records is usually taken at the end of the month. For example, if the number of delinquent records for January, February, and March is 200, 250, and 300, respectively, the average for the quarter is 250 delinquent records.

Concurrent and Retrospective Monitoring

Some medical staffs want to know, on a monthly basis, the number of records that did not have H&Ps dictated within 24 hours of admission and the number of patients who went to surgery without an H&P being on the record or being dictated. These statistics can be compiled concurrently by checking for the report as soon as the time frames have expired. They can also be compiled retrospectively, when the discharge record is received by the health information management department. Either way, the date of admission or surgery is checked against the date of dictation on the report. Reports not dictated within the time frames are reported to the medical staff for action. Keeping track of dictated reports can also be done by clerical staff in the transcription area.

Reporting Physicians Suspended

Also reported to the medical staff are the names of those physicians who were suspended because of delinquent medical records during the previous month. Again, a computerized system will usually provide a list (Figure 7.9) of the names. If using a manual system, you must be careful to ensure that the list is accurate.

```
CUMULATIVE SUSPENSION LIST          Jul 18, 2XXX              Page # 1
Doctors suspended 1 or more days between Jul 01, 2XXX  and Jul 31, 2XXX
------------------------------------------------------------------------
      Doctor Name          # Days Suspended        Status
------------------------------------------------------------------------

    EWING/JAMES                    8
    OBRIEN/PATRICK                 3
    MARTIN/EDWARD                  3
```

FIGURE 7.9 Computerized cumulative suspension list.

$\mathcal{M}$ANUAL DELINQUENT RECORD COUNT

Determining the number of incomplete/delinquent records using a manual system is extremely time-consuming. Departments often develop elaborate systems for determining the number of records. The most accurate system remains counting the actual records by discharge date. To do so, pick a date upon which the record becomes delinquent. For example, if the records are counted December 20 and the records become delinquent at fourteen days, any discharge prior to December 6 would be considered delinquent. One medical record clerk can then go through each record, calling off whether the chart is incomplete or delinquent while another medical record clerk makes hash marks on a sheet of paper. This system is not totally accurate because if a record is out of file, it cannot be counted. Therefore, consideration must be given to counting all records that are pulled for physicians and any incomplete records that have been pulled for other departments.

$\mathcal{S}$UMMARY

Working with physicians in the physician incomplete area requires knowing the medical record content and completion requirements in detail. The medical record clerk must be able to think quickly and clearly to best assist busy physicians.

$\mathcal{L}$EARNING ACTIVITIES

1. Explain how to determine if a record is incomplete or delinquent.
2. Differentiate between the different notification letters that are sent to physicians and their purpose.
3. What does the term *suspension because of delinquent records* mean to a physician?
4. Discuss the two different methods for filing incomplete records and the advantages and disadvantages of each.

5. True or False:

_____ Records should stay in the incomplete area after being pulled until the physician comes in to complete them, no matter how long it takes.

_____ Whenever a physician makes some sort of complaint, you should report it to your supervisor even if you have solved the problem.

_____ It is not necessary to know what items are on the deficiency slip because the indicator tags show the physician what needs to be completed.

_____ If a physician misses one signature but he or she has completed everything else, it is all right to mark the record complete.

_____ When dealing with an upset physician, always meet anger with anger.

_____ The physician files can be updated either manually or by computer whenever you have time or at least once a week.

6. Explain how to update the deficiency slip under the following circumstances:
   (a) All physicians have completed all items on a record.
   (b) Physician A has completed all items except one signature.
   (c) Physician B has dictated a discharge summary that has been returned from transcription.
   (d) Physician C has dictated an operative report.

7. With a fellow student, role-play the following situation in the physician incomplete area. Consider that Dr. Adams is extremely stressed. What should the medical record clerk say and do? Take turns playing both roles.

   Dr. Adams has arrived and begins to work on her incomplete records. After looking at the first record, she says, "I dictated this report the last time I was here. Why do you people always lose my dictation?"

8. Math problems:
   (a) General Hospital discharged an average of 480 patients per month last year. How many delinquent records is this hospital allowed to have on a monthly basis?
   (b) Mercy Hospital had an average of 1,500 discharges per month. How many delinquent records is this hospital allowed to have per month?

9. Retrieve the deficiency slips created in Exercise 6 of Chapter 6. Update them using the following information:

   Dr. S. Jones—Discharge summary has been dictated and received back from transcription.
   H&P is signed.
   All orders but one are signed.
   Progress note is signed.

   Dr. D. Martin—Consultation is signed.
   Procedure note is dictated and received from transcription.
   All orders are signed.

   Dr. T. Jones—Consultation is dictated and received from transcription.
   EKG is signed.
   All orders are signed.

   Dr. N. Owens—All orders are signed.
   Postanesthesia note is timed.

## CHAPTER 8

Confidentiality and Release of Information

VOCABULARY

Authorization Signed consent of the patient or his or her representative to release confidential information.

Certified copies Copies of the medical record that the custodian of records states, in writing, are true copies of the original record.

Conditions of admission A document signed by the patient at admission that specifies legal obligations of the patient and hospital, including agreement to pay bill and consent for simple procedures such as blood drawing and the like.

Confidentiality of Alcohol and Drug Abuse Patient Records Regulations Federal regulations that provide for maintaining the confidentiality of substance abuse treatment records.

Copy service A company that copies and mails records requested from a hospital.

Custodian of records The person designated with responsibility for maintaining and retrieving records in a business.

Freedom of Information Act (FOIA) Provides for access to government records.

HIV testing A blood test for the antibodies to human immunodeficiency virus. Presence of the antibodies indicates a possibility of later developing acquired immune deficiency syndrome (AIDS).

Health Insurance Portability and Accountability Act (HIPAA) Federal legislation that established standardization of coding and claims submission, security of computerized patient information, and privacy rules for all patient information.

Microfilm Greatly reduced images on film in the form of rolls or channels on index-sized cards (i.e., microfiche).

Preexisting condition A diagnosis known to have been treated prior to the implementation date of an insurance policy or the date of an accident.

Privacy Act of 1974 Provides regulations regarding confidentiality of records maintained on individuals.

Quash Annul or set aside.

Statute A law or established rule.

Subpoena An order by a court or attorney to appear at the specified time.

Subpoena duces tecum An order to appear in court or at a deposition with the records specified.

Witness fee A fee specified by state law to be paid a witness subpoenaed to appear in a court of law.

OBJECTIVES

When you have completed this chapter, you will be able to:

- Understand the importance of maintaining the confidentiality of patient records and information.
- Discuss the circumstances under which information may be released without patient consent.
- Discuss the circumstances under which information may be released only with patient consent.
- Discuss federal legislation regarding release of patient information.
- Discuss the impact of AIDS on the confidentiality of medical records.
- Demonstrate knowledge of release of information procedures for telephone requests, mail requests, and subpoenas.
- Discuss the differences in releasing general medical/surgical acute care records, substance abuse records, and psychiatric records.

*C*ONFIDENTIALITY OF THE MEDICAL RECORD

Employee Responsibility

The health information management department places a great deal of importance in maintaining the confidentiality and security of the medical record. Some might ask why, when it is only a record of the treatment a patient has received at a healthcare facility. But let us look at the type of information that can be found in a medical record. A physician may conduct an extensive physical exam when the patient is first admitted. At the same time, he or she obtains a history of the current illness, past medical history, family medical history, and psychosocial history. The physician may record that the patient has a past history of treatment for alcohol abuse or venereal disease. Or perhaps, under social history, the physician may record that the patient drinks a six-pack of beer every weekend. In psychiatric records, there may be documentation of child abuse, rape, or other aberrant sexual practices. This type of information is given to the physician with the understanding that it will be used only as a knowledge base in determining the correct treatment.

Discrimination

In our society, unfortunately, medical information has been and is used to discriminate against individuals. In the past, patients diagnosed with cancer or acquired immune deficiency syndrome (AIDS) lost their jobs because of their diagnoses. Health information management practitioners are responsible for ensuring that all information about a patient is released only to those persons who are authorized to receive it. The actual paper or computer record is considered the property of the healthcare facility; the information contained in the record is considered to be the property of the patient.

*R*ELEASE WITHOUT PATIENT CONSENT

Each hospital must determine, based on state and federal law, if there are certain items that can be released to anyone without the patient's express written consent. Generally, hospitals may release the patient's name, address, age, sex, and general condition (e.g., good, fair, critical). Some hospitals also release the nature of the illness, such as heart attack or fractured leg. By signing the hospital's conditions of admission form (which may be named differently in your facility), the patient is considered to have consented to any release of this information. If the patient does not want the information or any part of it released, he or she may so specify, in writing, and all hospital personnel must honor the patient's decision.

In federal hospitals, the only information that may be released without the patient's consent is verification of the patient's name and dates of treatment. Federal hospitals must adhere to the regulations of the Privacy Act, which will be discussed later.

Medical Emergencies

There are circumstances under which more specific medical information may be released without the patient's consent. If the patient is admitted to the emergency department of another facility, the treating physician may need to know the patient's past medical history, including any discharge medications. Under these circumstances, it is a standard practice to provide the necessary information to the other hospital and then document in the record the reason for the release, the date, the type of information released, the name of the person receiving the information, and the name of the person releasing the information.

Subpoenas

A **subpoena duces tecum** is a legal order to appear in court on a specified date with specified records. The consent of the patient is not required, although in some states the patient must be given notice, prior to service of the subpoena, that the records are being subpoenaed. This notice provides for a waiting period that allows the patient the opportunity to attempt to **quash** the **subpoena** or take legal action of his or her own. Records are usually subpoenaed because the patient is involved in a malpractice suit or, more commonly, an accident suit, where the patient's medical condition is pertinent to settlement of the case. The **custodian of records** (usually the director of health information management or a supervisor) must appear with the records when they are subpoenaed.

Law Enforcement

Occasionally, officials of law enforcement agencies will request access to a patient's medical record in conjunction with an investigation. An officer of the law is not automatically entitled to access. Depending on individual state law, information may be released only if the patient is in the act of committing a crime or presents a danger to himself or herself or others. The request must still be in writing and documentation regarding the circumstances of the release must be added to the record. Some states also have **statutes** regarding child abuse reporting that allow law enforcement personnel access to the child's or parent's record without the parent's consent.

Hospital Personnel

Earlier, we discussed the information that can be released after the patient signs the **conditions of admission.** Signing the conditions also authorizes the transmittal of information among hospital personnel so that they can perform their duties. For example, a nurse going off duty needs to communicate the patient's condition and treatment received to the next nurse taking over that patient's care. Or, the radiology department needs to know the **differential diagnosis** (the tentative diagnosis made before any tests are completed) to assist in the interpretation of the x-ray. Obviously, patients will not receive adequate treatment if hospital personnel are prevented from communicating confidential information among themselves. However, being a hospital employee or a member of the medical staff does not automatically entitle one to patient information. A telephone operator does not need to know the patient's diagnosis to do his or her job; similarly, a physician not treating a particular patient is not entitled to access that patient's medical record.

Medical Research

In Chapter 2, we discussed the use of the medical record in research. Physicians in the hospital setting may conduct research projects. This is especially true in teaching facilities that have residents and interns. In order to protect patient confidentiality, most hospitals have written policies regarding how research studies are conducted. Usually, the physician must submit a written request indicating the subject and reason for the study. For example, a physician may have a theory regarding the effect of aspirin in preventing heart attacks. The request is reviewed by a board of physicians for validity. Once approved by the board, the HIM department may then begin identifying the patients who fall under the study criteria and retrieving the records. The physician reviews the records, compiles data, and may eventually publish his or her findings in one of the medical journals. If the doctor publishes the finding, how is the patient's right to confidentiality maintained?

There are two methods. First, the physician may contact each patient and obtain written consent to use the information. The drawbacks to this method are obvious. Research studies can involve hundreds of patients. The process of tracking down all of them and obtaining consent could take months. And even if all patients could be located, not all of them may give consent. Valuable information could then be lost to the study, making definitive results unlikely.

The second method for maintaining patient confidentiality is more practical and the most commonly used in the hospital setting. As long as the physician does not use patient identifying information (i.e., name, address, medical record number), patient confidentiality is maintained. In his report, Dr. Smith can talk about Patient A, white male, age 65, and Patient B, black male, age 55, rather than Dan Jones, white male, age 65, and Robert Andrews, black male, age 55.

ℛ ELEASE REQUIRING PATIENT CONSENT

As we discussed earlier, the information that may be released without patient consent is minimal. If the patient's treatment is for a general medical or surgical condition, any information in the record may be released with written consent from the patient or his or her authorized representative (e.g., parent for minor, court appointed guardian, next of kin for deceased).

Physician Offices/Other Hospitals

Health information management departments receive requests daily from various third parties. Physician offices and other healthcare providers are frequent requesters.

When a patient sees a new physician for the first time, the physician will usually have the patient sign an **authorization** to obtain previous records. The records will give a more detailed history of the patient's illnesses and past treatment than the patient can usually supply. When a patient is admitted to a hospital with a diagnosis or symptoms that have been treated previously at a different hospital, the records will be requested so that the physician can see what treatment the patient received. This also ensures that diagnostic tests previously performed are not repeated unnecessarily.

Insurance Companies

Insurance companies submit a large number of requests for medical records. The information is used in determining whether a patient qualifies for a new insurance plan, be it life, health, or disability. A patient's health insurance company may request records to compare the documented diagnoses and procedures with the bill for hospital services.

With cost containment a priority, health insurance companies have increased the number of billing audits performed. An auditor will compare each item on the bill with documentation in the record. If the auditor cannot find the documentation (e.g., that a particular drug was administered), the insurance company will probably deny payment for that item. "If it isn't documented, it didn't happen." Depending on the contract the hospital has with the insurance company, a separate consent from the patient may be required prior to the occurrence of a billing audit.

Attorneys

Attorneys request medical records for a number of reasons, most commonly when a patient is involved in a third-party lawsuit. Perhaps the patient slipped and fell at a department store and then was treated at the hospital. The patient then contacted an attorney and decided to sue the store. The patient's attorney will request the records of all treatment received to prove the extent and cost of the injuries. The department store's attorney may request medical records documenting treatment prior to the injury, in an attempt to prove the injury was a **preexisting condition.** In either case, the consent of the patient is required unless the records are subpoenaed.

Records may also be requested by attorneys as evidence in criminal investigations.

*F*EDERAL PRIVACY ACT OF 1974

The **Privacy Act of 1974** (5 USC Section 552a) was enacted by the federal government in 1974. It provides regulations regarding the release of government records maintained on individuals, including medical records maintained at Department of Veterans Affairs and military hospitals. As discussed earlier, the Privacy Act requires written consent for the release of any information other than dates of treatment. This restriction also covers records that have been subpoenaed by a nonfederal court. The patient must give consent before the health information management department may respond to the subpoena.

*C*ONFIDENTIALITY OF SUBSTANCE ABUSE TREATMENT RECORDS

The treatment of drug/alcohol abuse is a sensitive issue in our society. Consequently, the **Confidentiality of Alcohol and Drug Abuse Patient Records law** (42 Code of

Federal Regulations, Chapter 1, Subchapter A, Part 2) was passed by Congress. This law sets forth regulations governing the confidentiality and release of drug and alcohol abuse treatment records. The regulations apply only to established treatment programs that are federally assisted. No information may be released without the patient's consent including acknowledgment of the patient's presence in the program. This makes sense; if a person is acknowledged to be a patient in a treatment program, his or her diagnosis is not difficult to determine.

Required Elements on Consent

The regulations also specify the elements that must be contained in the written consent, including the reason for the disclosure and a specified date on which the consent is no longer valid. When releasing information, hospitals must use a stamp on each set of copies that states that the records are released under federal regulations and may not be further disclosed without another written consent from the patient. The regulations do allow release without patient consent in certain cases. These include cases where child abuse is suspected or when the patient has threatened or participated in a crime against program facilities or personnel.

$\mathcal{H}$EALTH INSURANCE PORTABILITY AND ACCOUNTABILITY ACT (HIPAA)

The **Health Insurance Portability and Accountability Act (HIPAA)** of 1996 has an Administrative Simplification subtitle. The legislation mandates health care providers meet standards under three components: Transactions, Security, and Privacy. This is the first federal legislation that standardizes privacy of patient information and release of that information nationally. It establishes penalties for wrongful disclosure of individually identifiable health information.

Transactions

The transactions component requires that the process of coding and claims submission be standardized for all payers and providers. It replaces 400 versions of the UB92 and HCFA 1500 claims forms. Other eligibility, remittance advice, and benefit enrollment forms are also standardized. Claims must be submitted electronically and coding guidelines are mandated.

Security

The security component defines how to ensure privacy and protect confidentiality of protected health information. It requires providers to develop administrative procedures to ensure that security plans, policies, procedures, training, and contractual agreements exist. It also requires providers to develop physical safeguards of all computer media and devices. Technical security must be in place to provide specific authentication, authorization, access, and audit controls to prevent improper access to electronically stored information. Providers must also establish controls over their computer systems to avoid the risk of interception or alteration of data during electronic transmissions of data.

Privacy

The privacy component defines an individual's right to keep certain information to him- or herself with the understanding that the information will only be used or disclosed with his or her permission or as permitted by law. The patient has a right to receive a notice of Privacy Practice, request privacy protections, request restrictions on uses or disclosures, request confidential communications, access to inspect or copy information, amend information, and to accounting of disclosures except for those made to carry out treatment, payment, or operations of the provider. The legislation also requires that only the minimum information necessary be disclosed. It further mandates that each provider establish a Privacy Officer who has responsibility for insuring that all employees, physicians and volunteers are trained regarding the requirements of the privacy regulation.

The HIPAA requirements do not replace state law if the state law is already more stringent. However, this must be determined on a case-by-case basis. HIM departments will have even greater responsibility for releasing patient information properly.

CONFIDENTIALITY OF PSYCHIATRIC RECORDS

Because the treatment of psychiatric disorders often requires documentation of sensitive information, some states have passed protective legislation. These regulations usually are similar to the statutes regarding release of information for drug and alcohol abuse patients. A special consent is required to release the information, and instances in which information can be released without patient consent are very specific. HIPAA standardizes confidentiality and release requirements for psychiatric records.

PATIENT ACCESS TO RECORDS

Allowing a patient access to his or her record has long been debated. Some feel that the information is too technical for the average person to understand, thus leading to misinterpretation and possible detriment to the patient's well-being.

Among the states, legislation permitting patient access varies greatly. Some states allow hospitals to charge for copies of the record; others allow only review of the record with no copies. Still others allow copies, but the hospital must absorb the cost. Some specify a time frame for compliance with a request; others have no such specifications, allowing patients to demand same-day service. HIPAA standardizes a patient's right to access his or her record and/or amend it.

Freedom of Information Act

Under the **Freedom of Information Act (FOIA),** patients in federal hospitals may request access to their records. The law specifies the information to be included in the request, including the purpose for which the records will be used. Time frames for compliance and allowable charges for providing copies are also specified.

Under FOIA, a patient may also request amendment of the record. If the physician agrees to the amendment, the amended portion is then sent to all previous requesters of the record. If the physician does not approve the amendment, the patient may submit a statement regarding the information in question. The statement is made a part of the record and is sent with the record when it is released to a requester.

R RELEASE OF INFORMATION

We will now discuss specific procedures a medical record clerk might use to release information after becoming proficient in the various laws and regulations.

Telephone Requests

The most frequent requests for information received by a health information management department are telephone requests. They may come from physicians' offices, insurance companies, other hospitals, patients, and any number of persons or businesses. Following state law and federal regulations, the hospital will determine what items, if any, may be released without the patient's consent. These items may include the patient's name, address, age, sex, and general condition. If the telephone caller requests one of the items, the information may be released while the caller is still on the line. Verification of dates of treatment is also acceptable if the patient's treatment is not for a psychiatric condition or for substance abuse. For example, if an insurance company calls and states that the patient was admitted on August 6, it is acceptable to disclose that the patient was discharged on August 8. This information does not violate the patient's right to confidentiality, as the diagnosis is not revealed.

Physician offices often call to obtain information for use in their billing, including the patient's insurance information. When receiving such a request, take the requester's name, telephone number, and the physician's name. When ready with the requested information, always call back and verify that the requester is, in fact, working for that physician. It is possible that someone could fraudulently say he or she is from a physician's office to obtain patient information.

If a physician has not received his or her copy of a dictated report, laboratory result, or the patient's facesheet, his or her office will probably call the health information management department and request the copies. When taking such requests, write down the name of the physician, the telephone number, the name of the person making the request, and accurately describe the information that is needed. Obtaining dates that the patient was treated by the physician will help in locating the correct report.

Fax Requests

Every hospital has a policy regarding when records may be faxed to requestors. In most cases, records may be faxed only when they are needed for urgent or emergency patient care. Many hospitals interpret this to mean that the patient must be currently being treated in a hospital or physician's office.

Although faxing is very convenient for both the requestor and the clerk answering the request, it can be a very dangerous tool as far as patient confidentiality is concerned. If one digit of the fax number is entered incorrectly, the patient's record could end up printing in the local pizza shop instead of a physician's office. Most hospital policies require that the fax confirmation be filed in the medical record with the request. The confirmation shows the fax number the records went to and the number of pages received. If the department fax machine does not print confirmations, the clerk may be required to obtain a telephone confirmation.

Mail Requests

Requests received by mail are usually requests for actual copies of medical records and should be accompanied by a valid authorization. In answering this type of request from insurance companies, physician offices, attorneys, and the like, the following procedure should be followed.

*P*ROCEDURE FOR PROCESSING MAIL REQUESTS

1. *Valid Authorization.* Determine validity of each authorization by checking for the following information:
   a. Patient's name
   b. Authorization is directed specifically to the hospital
   c. Name and address of entity to receive information
   d. Dates and type of treatment records requested
   e. Date authorization expires
   f. Patient or authorized representative signature and date

2. *Alphabetical Order.* Place all requests in alphabetical order.

3. *Find Medical Record Numbers.* Check the master patient index (MPI) for each patient's name to find the medical record numbers.

4. *Determine if Requested Records Exist.* Check the MPI entry for each record requested to determine if there are records for the dates of treatment specified on the request. Remember that if the department has an older MPI on **microfilm,** it must also be checked if the request does not specify dates of treatment. If the patient cannot be identified with the information provided by the requester, set that particular request aside. For example, the request may ask for the records of Jose Garcia, but, in the MPI, there may be ten Jose Garcias. If the requester has not specified a date of treatment or provided a date of birth, it is impossible to identify the correct Jose Garcia.

5. *Put Requests in Terminal Digit Order.* Write the medical record numbers on the requests and put the requests in terminal digit order.

6. *Pull Records.* Pull the records. Remember that if the record is incomplete, it will probably be filed in a separate area.

7. *Compare Signatures.* Compare the signature on the authorization against the patient's signature on the Conditions of Admission form (Figure 8.1). If they appear to be the same, the records may be released. If they do not appear to be the same signature, check the actual record to ensure that it was the patient who signed the Conditions of Admission. In many cases the patient is too ill to sign, and the spouse or other family member will sign for him or her. It is also possible that because the patient is very ill, his or her signature may not appear the same as it does on the release authorization. If there is any doubt that the patient signed the authorization, refer the request and record to the supervisor for a decision.

   If the patient is not competent to sign or has expired, the legal guardian or next of kin may authorize release of information. This practice will vary from state to state.

8. *Copy Requested Records.* Copy only the portions of the record requested. If, for example, a physician's office requests only pathology reports, send only pathology reports. If the requester asks for all records, many departments send only dictated reports, abnormal laboratory results, and pathology reports. Some actually copy the entire record if it is requested. This policy will differ from department to department.

AUTHORIZATION FOR USE OR DISCLOSURE
OF MEDICAL INFORMATION

A. EXPLANATION:

This authorization for use or disclosure of medical information is being requested of you to comply with the terms of the Confidentiality of Medical Information Act of 1981, Section 56, et seq., California Civil Code.

B. AUTHORIZATION:

I hereby authorize ___*Mercy Medical Center*___

_____
(Name of Physician, Hospital or Health Care Provider)

to furnish to ___*Dr. Weber*___ medical records and information pertaining to medical history,
(Name of Requester)

mental or physical condition, services rendered, or treatment of ___*Debra Freeberg*___.
(Name of Patient)

This authorization is limited to the following medical records and type of information:
___*All Records*___

C. USES:

The requester may use the medical records and type of information authorized only for the following purposes:
___*Furthur Medical Care*___

D. DURATION:

This authorization shall become effective immediately and shall remain in effect until ___*1 – 1 – 2XXX*___.
(Date)

E. RESTRICTIONS:

I understand that requester may not further use or disclose the medical information unless another authorization is obtained from me or unless such use or disclosure is specifically required or permitted by law.

F. ADDITIONAL COPY:

I further understand that I have a right to receive a copy of this authorization upon my request. Copy requested and received: YES _____ NO __X__ Initial ___

G. SIGNATURE:

___*7 – 18 – 2XXX*___   Signed: ___*Debra Freeberg*___
    Date   *(Patient / Representative / Spouse* / Financially Responsible Party*)*

If signed by other than Patient, indicate relationship:

_____   _____
    Witness

* A spouse or financially responsible party may only authorize release of medical information for use in processing an application for the patient, as a spouse or dependent, for a health insurance plan or policy, a nonprofit hospital plan, a health care service plan or an employee benefit plan.

FIGURE 8.1 Check Authorization and Conditions of Admission to see if signatures match.

When pulling out the documents to be copied, ensure that they are from the correct episode of care. If the requester wants records from an admission in 2010 and records from 2008 are released, the patient's right to confidentiality has been violated because the patient has authorized only the release of the records requested. Often, records requested are incomplete at the time the request is received. Some hospitals choose to wait until the record is complete before releasing any information. Others release the information that is available and tell the requester that the other information (e.g., a discharge summary) is not available. The requester then has the option of working without the information or sending a second request at a later date. If a health information management department holds the request until the record is complete, it should have a policy

7. FINANCIAL OBLIGATIONS

The undersigned agrees, whether he/she signs as agent or as patient, that in return for the services to be rendered for the patient, the undersigned hereby individually obligates himself/herself to pay the account of the hospital in accordance with the regular rates and terms of the hospital. However, if the patient is eligible to receive benefits under a health care service plan with which this hospital has contracted, the patient shall not be obligated to pay for services covered under the plan which are paid for pursuant to the contract. If any excess funds remain after payment in full of the charges for services rendered for this hospital visit, the undersigned hereby authorizes the hospital to apply such excess funds toward any other outstanding account(s) which the patient may have with hospital for any prior services rendered and for which the undersigned is responsible. Should the patient's account become delinquent and be referred to an attorney or collection agency for collection, the undersigned shall pay actual attorney's fees and collection expenses. All delinquent accounts shall bear interest at the legal rate.

8. ASSIGNMENT OF INSURANCE OR HEALTH PLAN BENEFITS TO HOSPITAL

The undersigned authorizes, whether he/she signs as agent or as patient, direct payment to the hospital of any insurance benefits otherwise payable to or on behalf of the patient for this hospitalization or for these outpatient services, including emergency services if rendered, at a rate not to exceed the hospital's regular charges. It is agreed that payment to the hospital pursuant to this authorization by an insurance company or health plan shall discharge said insurance company or health plan of any and all obligations under the policy to the extent of such payment. It is understood by the undersigned that he/she is financially responsible for charges not covered by this assignment.

9. ASSIGNMENT OF INSURANCE OR HEALTH PLAN BENEFITS TO HOSPITAL-BASED PHYSICIANS

The undersigned authorizes, whether he/she signs as agent or as patient, direct payment to any hospital-based physician of any insurance or health plan benefits otherwise payable to or on behalf of the patient for professional services rendered during this hospitalization or for outpatient services, including emergency services if rendered, at a rate not to exceed such physician's regular charges. It is agreed that payment to such physician pursuant to this authorization by an insurance company or health plan shall discharge said insurance company or health plan of any and all obligations under the policy to the extent of such payment. It is understood by the undersigned that he/she is financially responsible for charges not covered by this assignment.

10. MEDICARE PATIENT'S RELEASE OF INFORMATION

I certify that the information given by me in applying for payment under Title XVIII of the Social Security Act is correct. I authorize release of any information needed to act on this request. I request that payment of authorized benefits be made in my behalf. I assign payment for the unpaid charges of the physician(s) for whom the hospital is authorized to bill in connection with its services. I understand I am responsible for any remaining balance not covered by other insurance.

The undersigned certifies that he/she has read the foregoing, received a copy thereof, and is the patient, the patient's legal representative, or is duly authorized by the patient as the patient's general agent to execute the above and accept its terms.

_____7 - 17 - 2XXX_____
Date

_____0800_____
Time

_____Sue Jones_____
Witness

_____Debra Freedman_____
Patient / Parent / Guardian / Conservator

If other than patient, indicate relationship: _____

Reason patient is unable to sign: _____

FINANCIAL RESPONSIBILITY AGREEMENT BY PERSON OTHER THAN THE PATIENT OR THE PATIENT'S LEGAL REPRESENTATIVE:

I agree to accept financial responsibility for services rendered to the patient and to accept the terms of the Financial Obligations (Paragraph 7) and Assignment of Insurance or Health Plan Benefits (Paragraphs 8 and 9) set forth above.

_____
Date

_____
Time

_____
Witness

_____
Financially Responsible Party

_____
Date

A COPY OF THIS DOCUMENT IS TO BE DELIVERED TO THE PATIENT AND ANY OTHER PERSON WHO SIGNS THIS DOCUMENT.

PATIENT NAME FREEBERG, DEBRA

MEDICAL RECORD NO. 06-40-75

PHYSICIAN ALLEN

ROOM # 502 A

FIGURE 8.1 Continued.

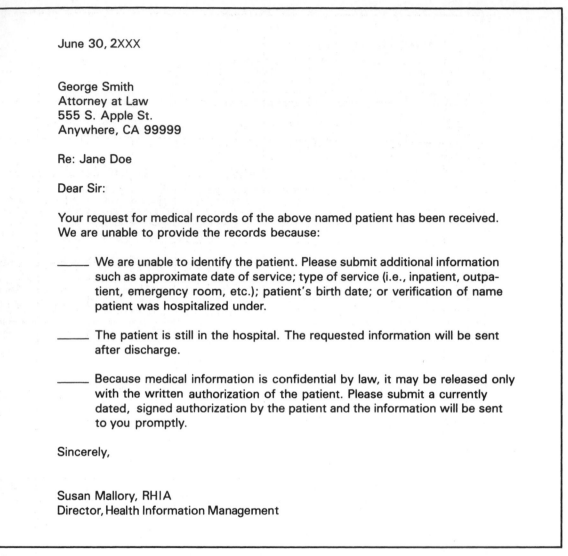

June 30, 2XXX

George Smith
Attorney at Law
555 S. Apple St.
Anywhere, CA 99999

Re: Jane Doe

Dear Sir:

Your request for medical records of the above named patient has been received.
We are unable to provide the records because:

_____ We are unable to identify the patient. Please submit additional information
such as approximate date of service; type of service (i.e., inpatient, outpatient, emergency room, etc.); patient's birth date; or verification of name
patient was hospitalized under.

_____ The patient is still in the hospital. The requested information will be sent
after discharge.

_____ Because medical information is confidential by law, it may be released only
with the written authorization of the patient. Please submit a currently
dated, signed authorization by the patient and the information will be sent
to you promptly.

Sincerely,

Susan Mallory, RHIA
Director, Health Information Management

FIGURE 8.2 Form letter used to answer requests for information on unidentifiable patients.

requiring that a letter be sent to the requester verifying that the request has
been received and explaining that it will not be answered until the record is
completed by all physicians.

9. *Bill for Copies.* Depending on state law, the department may be able to
charge for copies from certain requesters, such as insurance companies and
attorneys. Usually, in these states, a check for the copies will be sent with
the request. If a check is not received, a bill for services may be prepared.
The fee is usually based on a per hour retrieval charge billed in quarter-
hour increments, plus a specified fee per page.

10. *Mail the Requested Copies.* Place the requested copies, along with a copy
of the request and any bill that has been generated, in an envelope. Type
a label or handwrite legibly the address of the requester on the envelope.
Once all requests have been completed, batch the envelopes and process
them the same as other mail. This may involve actually taking them to
the mail room or placing them in an outbox in the department.

CORRESPONDENCE LOG

MEDICAL RECORD NUMBER:	PATIENT/NAME: LAST, FIRST		REQUESTING PARTY/ADDRESS:	INFO REQUESTED: (CIRCLE)	DATE REC'D	DATE SENT	INITIALS/NOTES
		Att Ins Med		FS DS HP CN OP PATH / PO PN ER LAB EKG XRAY / PT OT ST			
		Att Ins Med		FS DS HP CN OP PATH / PO PN ER LAB EKG RAY / PT OT ST			
		Att Ins Med		FS DS HP CN OP PATH / PO PN ER LAB EKG XRAY / PT OT ST			
		Att Ins Med		FS DS HP CN OP PATH / PO PN ER LAB EKG XRAY / PT OT ST			
		Att Ins Med		FS DS HP CN OP PATH / PO PN ER LAB EKG XRAY / PT OT ST			
		Att Ins Med		FS DS HP CN OP PATH / PO PN ER LAB EKG XRAY / PT OT ST			
		Att Ins Med		FS DS HP CN OP PATH / PO PN ER LAB EKG XRAY / PT OT ST			
		Att Ins Med		FS DS HP CN OP PATH / PO PN ER LAB EKG XRAY / PT OT ST			
		Att Ins		FS DS HP CN OP PATH / PO PN ER LAB EKG XRAY / PT OT ST			
		Att Ins Med		FS DS HP CN OP PATH / PO PN ER LAB EKG XRAY / PT OT ST			
		Att Ins Med		FS DS HP CN OP PATH / PO PN ER LAB EKG XRAY / PT OT ST			

PLEASE PRINT CLEARLY & BE SPECIFIC!

(Att=ATTORNEY, Ins=INSURANCE, Med=MEDICAL)

FIGURE 8.3 Manual correspondence log.

Requests with No Identified Record

To save time and duplication of effort, many health information management departments have a standard form letter (Figure 8.2) that is sent to requesters who have not provided enough information. The form letter usually contains a statement such as, "We have received your request regarding patient Jose Garcia. We are unable to process the request for the following reasons." This is followed by individual statements that can be checked off such as "We cannot identify the patient under the name given" and "Please provide date of birth, and dates and types of treatment." There is usually also an "Other" box in which special information not contained in other standard statements can be requested. On the form, type in the requester's name and address and check the correct box. Sign the letter if authorized to do so, or obtain a signature from the supervisor. If you are unable to locate a record, your department will probably have a standard "no record" letter that you will fill out and return with the request. Prepare an envelope with the requester's address, place the original request and the completed form letter in the envelope, and batch for mailing.

Correspondence Log

All requests for information should be entered into a log so that requests received can be tracked in case of inquiries. There are computer programs available to log correspondence requests. In a hospital with a low volume of requests, the log will probably consist of a manual entry notebook in which each request is entered as it is received. The log (Figure 8.3) should contain the patient's name, requester's name, the date the request was received, the date the information was released, and what information was released. If a "no record" letter is sent, this should be reflected in the log under type of information released.

> Once the record has been copied, the request should be filed in the area of the record designated by the department. The record should be refiled in permanent file or the incomplete file area.

$\mathcal{P}$ REPARING FOR COPY SERVICES

The use of **copy services** for release of information processing is widespread across the country. In hospitals utilizing a copy service, the procedure for releasing information begins the same as the procedure stated earlier for processing mail requests. Once the record has been pulled and the authorization verified, your job is, for the most part, finished. The copy service personnel are trained to read the request and determine which information in the record should be released. They do all of the copying, mailing of the record, and any billing that is allowed by state law. The copy service will indicate on the back of the request what information was released and the date, and file the request in the record. The correspondence log is usually also maintained by the copy service, either manually or on a computer system.

$\mathcal{R}$ ELEASE UNDER SUBPOENA

We have discussed previously that a subpoena is an order from an officer of the court, usually an attorney, to appear at a specified time and place. A subpoena duces

ATTORNEY OR PARTY WITHOUT ATTORNEY *(Name and Address)*:

TELEPHONE NO.:

FOR COURT USE ONLY

ATTORNEY FOR *(Name)*:

NAME OF COURT:

STREET ADDRESS:

MAILING ADDRESS:

CITY AND ZIP CODE:

BRANCH NAME:

PLAINTIFF/PETITIONER:

DEFENDANT/RESPONDENT:

CIVIL SUBPENA ☐ **Duces Tecum**

CASE NUMBER:

THE PEOPLE OF THE STATE OF CALIFORNIA, TO *(name)*:

1. **YOU ARE ORDERED TO APPEAR AS A WITNESS** in this action as follows unless you make a special agreement with the person named in item 3:

   a. Date: Time: Dept./Div.:   Room.:

   b. Address:

2. **AND YOU ARE**

   a. ☐ ordered to appear in person.

   b. ☐ not required to appear in person if you produce a true, legible, and durable copy of the records described in the accompanying affidavit as follows: (1) place the copy of the records in an envelope (or other wrapper) and seal it; (2) attach a copy of this subpena to the envelope or write on the envelope the case name and number, name of the witness and date and time from item 1 above; (3) place this first envelope in an outer envelope or wrapper, seal it, and mail it to the clerk of the court at the address in item 1.

   c. ☐ ordered to appear in person and to produce the records described in the accompanying affidavit. The personal attendance of the custodian of records or other qualified witness and the production of the original records is required by this subpena. The procedure authorized pursuant to subdivision (b) of section 1560, and sections 1561 and 1562, of the Evidence Code will not be deemed sufficient compliance with this subpena.

3. **IF YOU HAVE ANY QUESTIONS ABOUT WITNESS FEES OR THE TIME OR DATE FOR YOU TO APPEAR, OR IF YOU WANT TO BE CERTAIN THAT YOUR PRESENCE IS REQUIRED, CONTACT THE ATTORNEY REQUESTING THIS SUBPENA, NAMED ABOVE, OR THE FOLLOWING PERSON, BEFORE THE DATE ON WHICH YOU ARE TO APPEAR:**

   a. Name: b. Telephone number:

4. **Witness Fees:** You are entitled to witness fees and mileage actually traveled both ways, as provided by law, if you request them at the time of service. You may request them before your scheduled appearance from the person named in item 3.

5. You are ordered to appear in this civil matter in your capacity as a peace officer or other person described in Government Code section 68097.1.

   Date: Clerk, by _____ , Deputy

DISOBEDIENCE OF THIS SUBPENA MAY BE PUNISHED AS CONTEMPT BY THIS COURT. YOU WILL ALSO BE LIABLE FOR THE SUM OF FIVE HUNDRED DOLLARS AND ALL DAMAGES RESULTING FROM YOUR FAILURE TO OBEY.

Date issued:

....
(TYPE OR PRINT NAME)

▶ _____
(SIGNATURE OF PERSON ISSUING SUBPENA)

_____
(TITLE)

(See reverse for proof of service)

Form Adopted by Rule 982
Judicial Council of California
982(a)(15) [Rev. July 1, 1987]

CIVIL SUBPENA

Code of Civil Procedure, §§ 1985, 1986, 1987

FIGURE 8.4 Example of a subpoena duces tecum.

tecum (Figure 8.4) is an order to appear with the records at a specified time and place. Subpoenas should be processed as soon as they are received. The following items should be checked on the subpoena before accepting service.

Accepting the Subpoena

1. The subpoena should be made out to the custodian of records with the hospital's name. Never accept a subpoena that is issued to a specific person, such as a physician or the hospital administrator. The person serving the subpoena should be directed to the correct office in the hospital or to the physician's office.

2. Check the date for which the custodian is ordered to appear. Many states have laws specifying the amount of time prior to appearance that the subpoena must be served. If the time limit is not met, service of the subpoena can be refused. Reasons for refusing service will be contained in a department policy that should be discussed with the director.

3. Check that the patient's name and dates of treatment records being requested are specified. If no such information is specified, ask for it from the person serving the subpoena, even though he or she may not have the information. This is not grounds for refusing service.

4. Write down the date and time of service and the person serving the subpoena (e.g., process server or marshall) at the top of the subpoena.

5. Some states require that the patient be notified that the records are being subpoenaed. If so, there will be a time frame for notification to the patient, and there should be a form attached to the subpoena that states the date on which the patient was informed. If the time frame specified by law has not been met, accept the subpoena and then notify the issuing attorney, in writing if necessary, why it will not be honored.

6. Most states have laws regarding **witness fees.** In some, if the fee is not demanded at the time the subpoena is served, the attorney is not required to pay later. If this is the case, inquire whether the process server has the check. If he or she does not, demand the check. Note at the top of the subpoena that the fee was asked for, whether it was received, and the amount. Fees for appearance will differ from state to state and some will depend on whether the custodian of records is actually required to appear. In some states, certified copies of the record are admissible as evidence in a court of law and the fee is then based on retrieval time plus a fee per page of the record.

Processing the Subpoena

Once the subpoena has been accepted, process it using the following procedure.

1. *Check MPI for Medical Record Number.* Check the MPI to determine the patient's medical record number and determine if the requested records exist. If the hospital has departments that keep separate records, such as radiology or physical therapy, remember that there may not be an MPI card. These department records must also be produced when subpoenaed.

2. *Pull the Record.* If an MPI entry is located, pull the record. Examine the subpoena carefully. Many subpoenas request not only medical records but also copies of the bill sent to the patient by the hospital business office. If this is the case, provide the patient number to the business office so that the staff can pull the records and make a copy of the bill to be included with the record.

    Once a determination has been made that the records specified on the subpoena are available, the attending physician may be notified by letter or telephone that the record has been subpoenaed. This is done as a courtesy so that the physician knows that the record is involved in a lawsuit.

3. *Copy the Record.* Copy the entire record. Make sure that all laboratory reports that are shingled can be read legibly when copied. If one report has been placed on the sheet so that it covers up another, they will have to be taken apart so that all results can be read. Some departments have a policy requiring that each page of the record be numbered before being copied. However, because of time and staffing constraints, this is not generally done.

4. *Complete Affidavit.* When the record is copied, complete the affidavit and have the custodian of records sign it. The affidavit (Figure 8.5) is a document signed by the custodian of records that states that the enclosed copies are true copies of the original record and that the documentation was made in the record by hospital employees at or near the time of the stated events.

AFFIDAVIT OF CUSTODIAN OF MEDICAL RECORDS

I, _____,
                     (Custodian of Medical Records)
declare that:

    (a) I am the duly authorized custodian of the medical records of _____ Hospital and have the authority to certify said records; and

    (b) The copy of the medical records attached to this Affidavit is a true copy of all the records described in the subpoena duces tecum; and

    (c) The records were prepared by the personnel of the hospital, staff physicians, or persons acting under the control of either, in the ordinary course of Hospital business at or near the time of the act, condition or event.

    I declare under penalty of perjury that the foregoing is true and correct.

_____   _____
Date   **(Signature of Affiant)**

FIGURE 8.5 Affidavit attached to certified record copies.

```
CASE:      Doe v. Jones
DATE:      July 1, 2XXX
WITNESS:   Mercy Medical Center
CASE NO.:  46734
```

FIGURE 8.6 Example of documentation on inner envelope when sending certified records to court.

5. *Prepare Envelopes.* Prepare the mailing envelope. On the outside (Figure 8.6) type the name of the case (e.g., *Woods* v. *Waters*) and the date of the subpoena. This is the date the witness must appear as specified on the subpoena. On the next line, type "Witness:" followed by the name of the hospital. The case number should also be typed on the envelope. This is a number assigned by the court and can be found on the subpoena. Seal the affidavit and the copies in the envelope. Place the first envelope in a larger envelope which has been addressed either to the court or to the attorney who subpoenaed the records. The purpose for using double envelopes is to ensure that the records are not tampered with before they are entered as evidence.

6. *Prepare Certified Mail Documentation.* Prepare a certified domestic mail return receipt to be placed on the envelope. The certified number will be obtained from the receipt for certified mail, which must also be completed (Figure 8.7). Attach the return receipt on the back of the envelope. Detach the certified number from the receipt for certified mail and place the certified number on the front of the envelope just to the left of the return address. It is a good idea to use tape to make sure that the certified number sticks.

7. *File Subpoena.* Attach the receipt to the subpoena. Then write the date the records were mailed on the subpoena, and initial. File the subpoena in the designated area of the record, and refile the record in the permanent file or the incomplete file area.

*R*ELEASE OF SUBSTANCE ABUSE TREATMENT RECORDS

Consent Form

In hospitals with federally funded substance abuse (i.e., alcohol or drug) treatment programs, federal law requires that, prior to release of the records, the patient sign a special consent form (Figure 8.8). The general consent form used for all other releases is not acceptable for these types of records. The special consent must specify the type of records to be released, the purpose for the release, and a date upon which the consent is no longer valid. If the patient does not specify a date, the consent is valid only until the information requested has been released. The procedure for identifying and copying the record is the same as that used for general release of information.

SENDER: Complete items 1 and 2 when additional services are desired, and complete items 3 and 4.

Put your address in the "RETURN TO" Space on the reverse side. Failure to do this will prevent this card from being returned to you. <u>The return receipt fee will provide you the name of the person delivered to and the date of delivery</u>. For additional fees the following services are available. Consult postmaster for fees and check box(es) for additional service(s) requested.

1. ☐ Show to whom delivered, date, and addressee's address.   2. ☐ Restricted Delivery
   ↑*(Extra charge)*↑   ↑*(Extra charge)*↑

3. Article Addressed to:

Clerk of the Court
Anywhere Municipal Court
623 Olive St
Anywhere, CA 99999

4. Article Number
P 884 311 424

Type of Service:
☐ Registered   ☐ Insured
☒ Certified   ☐ COD
☐ Express Mail

Always obtain signature of addressee or agent and <u>DATE DELIVERED</u>.

5. Signature — Addressee
X

6. Signature — Agent
X

7. Date of Delivery

8. Addressee's Address *(ONLY if requested and fee paid)*

PS Form **3811**, Mar. 1987   ★ U.S.G.P.O. 1987-178-268   **DOMESTIC RETURN RECEIPT**

P 884 311 424

RECEIPT FOR CERTIFIED MAIL
NO INSURANCE COVERAGE PROVIDED
NOT FOR INTERNATIONAL MAIL
(See Reverse)

Sent to *Clerk of Ct, Anywhere Municipal CA*

Street and No. *623 Olive St.*

P.O., State and ZIP Code *Anywhere, CA 99999*

Postage	$
Certified Fee	
Special Delivery Fee	
Restricted Delivery Fee	
Return Receipt showing to whom and Date Delivered	
Return Receipt showing to whom, Date, and Address of Delivery	
TOTAL Postage and Fees	$
Postmark or Date	

PS Form 3800, June 1985

Fold at line over top of envelope to the right of the return address

CERTIFIED

P 884 311 424

MAIL

FIGURE 8.7 A completed domestic mail return receipt and a receipt for certified mail.

Confidentiality Statement

Once the records are ready to be mailed, the law requires that the following statement be stamped on each set of copies:

> This information has been disclosed to you from records protected by federal confidentiality rules (42 CFR Part 2). The Federal rules prohibit you from making any further disclosure of this information unless further disclosure is expressly permitted by the written consent of the person to whom it pertains or as otherwise permitted by 42 CFR Part 2. A general authorization for the release of medical or other information is NOT sufficient for this purpose. The federal rules restrict any use of the information to criminally investigate or prosecute any alcohol or drug abuse patient.

This statement reminds the person receiving the records that they have been released under federal law and that they may not be further released to any other person without another written consent from the patient. For example, if the patient had signed a consent allowing the release of the records to a physician, that physician could not then release those same records to a second physician without first obtaining another written consent.

Records Pertaining to Other Persons

When releasing substance abuse records, care should be taken not to release any information that pertains to persons other than the patient. Because family counseling is often a part of substance abuse treatment, the records may contain sensitive information about the patient's relationship with family members. Legally, the patient can only consent to information about himself or herself being released.

Subpoenas

A department that receives a subpoena for substance abuse records has two options. If the documentation relating to the substance abuse treatment is a minor part of the record, that portion of the record may be omitted from the information released. The court or attorney who has subpoenaed the records is then told that a portion of the record is being omitted because it is protected by federal law. If the entire record is related to substance abuse treatment, the health information management department cannot release the records unless ordered to do so by a judge. The judge actually has to review the record and make a determination about whether release of the records under the subpoena would be harmful to the patient. If the judge decides that the release would not be harmful to the patient, he or she may issue a court order to the custodian of records to release the information. This procedure must be followed even if the patient gives his or her consent to the release. The procedures for processing the subpoenaed record would be the same as previously discussed.

Telephone Requests

The federal Confidentiality of Alcohol and Drug Abuse Patient Records regulations state that a hospital cannot acknowledge the presence of a patient being treated for substance abuse because such an acknowledgment would indicate the type of treat-

CONSENT FOR RELEASE OF ALCOHOL OR DRUG ABUSE PATIENT INFORMATION OR RECORDS*

I hereby authorize _____

(Name of Organization Conducting Program)

to disclose records obtained in the course of the diagnosis and treatment of _____

_____

(Name of Patient)

for alcohol and/or drug abuse to _____ .

(Name of Person or Organization to Which Disclosure Is Made)

The disclosure of records authorized herein is required for the following purpose: _____

_____ ;

and such disclosure shall be limited to the following specific types of information: _____

_____

_____

This consent is subject to revocation by the undersigned at any time except to the extent that action has been taken in reliance hereon, and if not earlier revoked, it shall terminate on _____

_____

(Date, Event, or Condition)

without express revocation.

_____   _____
Dated   *(Patient, Parent, Guardian, or Authorized Representative of Patient)*

If signed by other than patient, indicate relationship:

_____

*NOTE: Patient consent forms for the release of records to central registries or in connection with criminal justice referrals must meet certain additional requirements. (See 42 C.F.R. Sections 2.34 and 2.35.)

FIGURE 8.8 Consent form to release drug/alcohol abuse records.

ment and violate the patient's right to confidentiality. Telephone requests for information about a patient known to be in the hospital substance abuse unit should receive a noncommittal response as to whether the person is a patient. The call should then be transferred to the substance abuse treatment unit. If the caller says that he or she knows the patient is in the unit, transfer the call to the unit without acknowledging that the patient is in the hospital. Such a call might proceed as follows: "This is Jane Doe. I'd like to speak to David Doe, please." The medical record clerk replies, "I'm sorry, I have no knowledge of that person being a patient. Let me transfer you to someone who may be able to help." "He's a patient on the alcohol treatment unit," says Jane Doe. "I'll transfer you to that unit," says the medical record clerk.

$\mathcal{R}$ ELEASE OF PSYCHIATRIC RECORDS

As in substance abuse records, psychiatric records often contain extremely confidential information about the patient and family members. Some states—for example, California and Oklahoma—have laws similar to the federal alcohol and drug abuse regulations and require a special consent (Figure 8.9) from the patient before psychiatric records may be released. Others have no specific laws. Hospitals in states without specific laws often pattern the release of psychiatric information after the federal alcohol and drug abuse regulations. When releasing psychiatric records, information pertaining to persons other than the patient should not be released without those persons' specific consent.

$\mathcal{R}$ ELEASE OF AIDS RECORDS

In those states that have laws regarding confidentiality of **human immunodeficiency virus (HIV) antibody testing**, health information management departments have clear-cut guidelines as to what information can or cannot be released. Persons with a positive HIV test are considered to be at risk for later developing acquired immune deficiency syndrome (AIDS). The laws in California, Colorado, Florida, and Oklahoma are similar in that they require that the patient be counseled regarding the meaning of a positive or negative test result and that the patient sign a consent prior to the blood drawing.

Usually, the test results are considered extremely confidential and cannot be released to any third party without a special written consent (Figure 8.10) from the patient. In those states without protective law, the release of information regarding HIV testing and the actual diagnosis of AIDS is likely to be determined by medical staff and hospital policy, as well as the community standard.

CONSENT FOR RELEASE OF INFORMATION OR RECORDS UNDER LANTERMAN-PETRIS-SHORT ACT

I, _____ hereby authorize _____
　　　　Name of Patient　　　　　　　　　　　　　　　　　　　Name of Administrator of Program

to disclose information and records obtained in the course of my diagnosis and treatment to

_____
　　　　　　　　　Name of Person or Organization to Which Disclosure Is Made

The disclosure of information and records authorized herein is required for the following purpose:

_____

Such disclosure shall be limited to the following specific types of information:

_____

_____　　　_____
　　　　　　Dated　　　　　　　　　　　　　　　　　　　　　　Patient

_____
　　　　　　Witness

The undersigned, the physician, licensed psychologist, or social worker with a masters degree in social work, who is in charge of the patient, hereby (approves) (disapproves) the release of information and records to the party specified above. If disclosure is disapproved, give reasons below. Also note below any restrictions on the release of records. (**Note:** No approval is required for release to the patient's attorney.)

_____

_____

_____

_____　　_____ , 　_____
　　　Date　　　　　　　　　Physician/Psychologist/Social Worker　　　　　　　　Degree

Welfare & Institutions Code Section 5328.7

FIGURE 8.9 Consent used in California for release of psychiatric information.

AUTHORIZATION FOR DISCLOSURE OF THE RESULTS OF THE HIV ANTIBODY BLOOD TEST

Patient: _____

A. EXPLANATION

This authorization for use or disclosure of the results of a blood test to detect antibodies to the Human Immunodeficiency Virus (HIV), the probable causative agent of Acquired Immune Deficiency Syndrome (AIDS), is being requested of you to comply with the terms of the Confidentiality of Medical Information Act, Civil Code Section 56, et seq. and Health and Safety Code Section 199.21(g).

B. AUTHORIZATION

I hereby authorize _____
                                                    (Name of Physician, Hospital or Health Care Provider)

to furnish to _____
                                                    (Name or Title of Person Who Is to Receive Results)

the results of the blood test for antibodies to the HIV.

C. USES

The requester may use the information for any purpose, subject only to the following limitations: _____

_____

D. DURATION

This authorization shall become effective immediately and shall remain in effect indefinitely, or until _____,

_____ , whichever is shorter.

E. RESTRICTIONS

I understand that the requestor may not further use or disclose the medical information unless another authorization is obtained from me or unless such use or disclosure is specifically required or permitted by law.

F. ADDITIONAL COPY

I further understand that I have a right to receive a copy of this authorization upon my request.

Copy requested and received: _____ Yes _____No   Initial _____

Date: _____ , _____   _____
                                                                              Signature

Time: _____   If signed by other than patient, give relationship:*

Witness: _____   _____
                                                                              Legal Relationship to Patient

FIGURE 8.10 California consent form for release of HIV test results.

SUMMARY

Maintaining the confidentiality of patient information and medical records is the responsibility of each hospital employee, but it is particularly the responsibility of the medical records/HIM clerk. The medical records/HIM clerk must know the applicable state and federal regulations regarding release of information and apply them to the requests for information received daily in the health information management department.

LEARNING ACTIVITIES

1. True or False (if false, explain why):

   __ All information about a patient may be released at any time.
   __ Response to a subpoena requires patient consent.
   __ All hospital employees have the responsibility for protecting patient information.
   __ All hospital employees have the right to know the patient's diagnosis.
   __ Some states allow patients access to their medical records.
   __ Name, address, age, sex, and general condition can be released without patient consent.
   __ The FOIA is a federal regulation governing all patient records.
   __ Records should be faxed anytime a request for release of information is received.
   __ HIPAA allows a patient to request amendment of his or her record.
   __ HIPAA replaces all state laws related to confidentiality of patient records.

2. If release requires written patient consent, mark "Y"; if not, mark "N."

   __ A law enforcement investigation
   __ Insurance company for bill payment
   __ Drug/alcohol treatment records
   __ Attorney
   __ Subpoena served on a nonfederal hospital
   __ Medical emergency
   __ Research projects
   __ Physicians/other hospitals

3. Discuss the procedure for releasing information over the telephone, including substance abuse treatment information.

4. Which items should be checked for before accepting service of the subpoena?

5. What items should the medical records/HIM clerk document on the subpoena at the time of service?

6. In answering mail requests, number the following steps in the order that they would be performed.

___ Write the medical record numbers on the requests and put them in terminal digit order.

___ Check the MPI for each patient's name to find the medical record numbers.

___ Check the signature on the authorization against the patient's signature on the Condition of Admission.

___ Copy only the portions of the record requested.

___ Prepare a bill for services, if appropriate.

___ Pull the records.

___ Check each request for the patient's name.

___ Check the MPI entry for dates of treatment requested.

___ Mail the requested copies.

7. What procedures should be followed if the record specified on an authorization or a subpoena cannot be located?

8. Explain the difference between releasing general medical/surgical acute care records and substance abuse/psychiatric records.

9. You are the medical records/HIM clerk answering telephone requests for information. In each of the following conversations, what would be your reply?

(a) "This is Pam Beale from Dr. Daniel Jones's office. I need a facesheet and the operative report for patient Janice Anderson."

(b) "This is Sue Chang from Acme Insurance. I need to obtain the discharge date for patient David Goldstein, admitted 6/3/90."

(c) "This is Ray Warren. My wife was a patient there, and I need to get copies of her record."

(d) "This is Geraldo Ramirez from *The Examiner*. I'm doing a story on the car accident this morning involving Jane Doe. What's her diagnosis?"

(e) "This is Sandy Miller. I'd like to speak to John Doe. He's being treated on your alcohol unit."

## CHAPTER 9

Other Medical Records/ Health Information Clerk Functions

Amendment of birth certificate Filing a change with the state because information on the original birth certificate was incorrect or omitted.

Dictation system The recorders on which physicians dictate reports and the management software that lists each dictation job by date, time, dictator, report type, and so forth.

Paternity declaration A legal document used to establish paternity of a child when the mother and father are not married to each other.

Registration of birth Completing the required birth certificate form and filing it with the state department of health.

Transcription log A list of all dictation recorded by date received and transcribed, type of report, patient name, and physician dictating.

Transcription system The computers on which transcriptionists produce reports and the word processing software that assists them.

OBJECTIVES

When you have completed this chapter, you will be able to:

- Describe the procedure for obtaining birth certificate information and processing the birth certificate.
- Discuss the purpose for obtaining a Paternity Declaration.
- Demonstrate knowledge of transcription clerk duties.
- Discuss possible medical records/health information clerk functions under the titles cancer registry clerk, optical imaging clerk, outpatient clinic clerk, and case management clerk.

In this chapter we will examine various other functions that may be performed by a medical records/HIM clerk either in the HIM department or as an employee of another hospital department. These include birth certificate clerk, transcription clerk, case management clerk, cancer registry clerk, outpatient clinic clerk, and optical imaging clerk.

$\mathcal{B}$IRTH CERTIFICATES

Legal Requirements

The **registration of birth** is a requirement in every state. The function of obtaining birth certificate information, completing the certificate, and submitting it to the state for registration usually is performed in the health information management department. In some hospitals the obstetrical department will handle registration. In a hospital with a large volume of births each month, there may be several clerks whose sole function is processing birth certificates. In a hospital with a lower birth volume, the HIM department may have a medical records/HIM clerk who processes birth certificates as one of his or her duties.

The birth certificate, itself, is a legal document necessary to prove citizenship, to apply for a social security number, and to obtain a passport. The variety of information that is collected on a birth certificate is determined by each state government. The federal government requires that this information be reviewed and updated periodically. All birth certificates contain demographic information about the parents and information regarding the circumstances of the birth. In Hawaii, extensive family history is recorded. Other states, including California (Figure 9.1), require collection of detailed information including number of prenatal visits, pregnancy history, parents' occupations, and number of years of education for each parent. In Wisconsin, the detailed information (Figure 9.2) is collected separately from the actual birth certificate. The data are kept confidential and are used in collection of statewide statistics. Only information pertaining to the birth and identification of parents is released when a certified birth certificate is requested. This would include the baby's full name, date of birth, time of birth, name and signature of the physician delivering the baby, both parents' names (including mother's maiden name), the parents' dates of birth, and the signature of one parent.

$\mathcal{P}$ROCESSING OF CERTIFICATE

Worksheet

The most common method for obtaining birth certificate information is for the birth certificate clerk to interview the patient. The health information management department usually has a worksheet on which to write down the information, or it may be entered directly into a computer. The worksheet will probably be similar in format to the actual birth certificate form. In Wisconsin, the worksheet (Figure 9.3) is signed by the parent and the information is transmitted to the state electronically. When writing down names it is important that the parent, or informant, be asked to spell them. Once a birth certificate has been registered, the original can never be changed. Changes to the original information may be filed on an **amendment.** If an amendment is filed, a copy of the amendment is sent along whenever a copy of the original birth certificate is requested.

Accuracy

Accuracy is extremely important if you are producing a birth certificate using a typewriter. Because it is a legal document, there can be no use of opaquing or other forms of correction. However, typewriters with correction tape may be used if the correction cannot be seen. If, however, it is obvious that an error was made and corrected,

CERTIFICATE OF LIVE BIRTH
STATE OF CALIFORNIA
USE BLACK INK ONLY

	STATE FILE NUMBER		LOCAL REGISTRATION DISTRICT AND CERTIFICATE NUMBER

THIS CHILD	1A. NAME OF CHILD — FIRST (GIVEN)	1B. MIDDLE	1C. LAST (FAMILY)
	2. SEX	3A. THIS BIRTH, SINGLE, TWIN, ETC.	3B. IF MULTIPLE, THIS CHILD 1ST, 2ND, ETC.	4A. DATE OF BIRTH — MM/DD/CCYY	4B. HOUR — (24 HOUR CLOCK TIME)

PLACE OF BIRTH	5A. PLACE OF BIRTH — NAME OF HOSPITAL OR FACILITY		5B. STREET ADDRESS — STREET, NUMBER, OR LOCATION
	5C. CITY	5D. COUNTY	5E. PLANNED PLACE OF BIRTH

FATHER OF CHILD	6A. NAME OF FATHER — FIRST (GIVEN)	6B. MIDDLE	6C. LAST (FAMILY)	7. STATE OF BIRTH	8. DATE OF BIRTH
MOTHER OF CHILD	9A. NAME OF MOTHER — FIRST (GIVEN)	9B. MIDDLE	9C. LAST (MAIDEN)	10. STATE OF BIRTH	11. DATE OF BIRTH

INFORMANT CERTIFICATION	I CERTIFY THAT I HAVE REVIEWED THE STATED INFORMATION AND THAT IT IS TRUE AND CORRECT TO THE BEST OF MY KNOWLEDGE.	12A. PARENT OR OTHER INFORMANT — SIGNATURE	12B. RELATIONSHIP TO CHILD	12C. DATE SIGNED
CERTIFICATION OF BIRTH	I CERTIFY THAT THE CHILD WAS BORN ALIVE AT THE DATE, HOUR AND PLACE STATED.	13A. ATTENDANT OR CERTIFIER — SIGNATURE — DEGREE OR TITLE	13B. LICENSE NUMBER	13C. DATE SIGNED
	13D. TYPED NAME, TITLE AND MAILING ADDRESS OF ATTENDANT		14. TYPED NAME AND TITLE OF CERTIFIER IF OTHER THAN ATTENDANT	

LOCAL REGISTRAR	15A. DATE OF DEATH	15B. STATE FILE NO. (STATE USE ONLY)	16. LOCAL REGISTRAR — SIGNATURE	17. DATE ACCEPTED FOR REGISTRATION

CONFIDENTIAL INFORMATION FOR PUBLIC HEALTH USE ONLY

FATHER	18. RACE	19. HISPANIC	20A. USUAL OCCUPATION	20B. USUAL KIND OF BUSINESS OR INDUSTRY	20C. EDUCATION - YRS COMPLETED
	21. RACE	22. HISPANIC	23A. USUAL OCCUPATION	23B. USUAL KIND OF BUSINESS OR INDUSTRY	23C. EDUCATION - YRS COMPLETED
MOTHER	24A. RESIDENCE — STREET, NUMBER, OR LOCATION			24B. COUNTY	
	24C. CITY			24D. STATE	24E. ZIP CODE

MEDICAL DATA	25A. DATE LAST NORMAL MENSES BEGAN	25B. MONTH PRENATAL CARE BEGAN	25C. NUMBER OF PRENATAL VISITS	27. PREGNANCY HISTORY (COMPLETE EACH SECTION)		

ENTER THE APPROPRIATE CODE(S) FOR ITEMS 25D AND 28A THRU 31 FROM THE VS10A SUPPLEMENTAL WORKSHEET.

27. PREGNANCY HISTORY (COMPLETE EACH SECTION)

LIVE BIRTHS (DO NOT COUNT THIS CHILD)		OTHER TERMINATIONS (EXCLUDE INDUCED ABORTIONS)	
NOW LIVING	NOW DEAD	BEFORE 20 WEEKS	AFTER 20 WEEKS
A	B	D	E

25D. PRINCIPAL SOURCE OF PAYMENT FOR PRENATAL CARE	26. BIRTHWEIGHT	28A. METHOD OF DELIVERY

28B. EXPECTED PRINCIPAL SOURCE OF PAYMENT FOR DELIVERY	29. COMPLICATIONS AND PROCEDURES OF PREGNANCY AND CONCURRENT ILLNESSES	DATE OF LAST LIVE BIRTH (C)	DATE OF LAST OTHER TERMINATION (F)

30. COMPLICATIONS AND PROCEDURES OF LABOR AND DELIVERY	31. ABNORMAL CONDITIONS AND CLINICAL PROCEDURES RELATED TO THE NEWBORN

A.	B.	C.	D.	E.	F.	CENSUS TRACT	32. FATHER'S SOCIAL SECURITY NO.	33. MOTHER'S SOCIAL SECURITY NO.

VS 10D (REV. 5/97)

PRIVACY NOTIFICATION

This information is collected by the State of California, Department of Health Services, Office of Vital Records, 304 S Street, Sacramento, CA 95814, telephone number (916) 445-2684. The information is required by Division 9 of the Health and Safety Code. This record is open to public access except where prohibited by statute. Every element on this form, except items 18 through 23C, 32, and 33, is mandatory. Failure to comply is a misdemeanor. The principal purposes of this record are to: 1) Establish a legal record of each vital event; 2) Provide certified copies for personal use; 3) Furnish information for demographic and epidemiological studies; and 4) Supply data to the National Center for Health Statistics for federal reports. Items 32 and 33 are included pursuant to Section 102425 (b) (14) of the Health and Safety Code, and may be used for child support enforcement purposes.

Definition of Live Birth

"Live Birth" means the complete expulsion or extraction from its mother of a product of conception (irrespective of duration of pregnancy) which, after such separation, breathes or shows any other evidence of life such as beating of the heart, pulsation of the umbilical cord, or definite movement of voluntary muscles, whether or not the umbilical cord has been cut or the placenta is attached.

97 90466

FIGURE 9.1 California birth certificate.

Data Validator _____

Processor _____

Mother's Name _____ / _____ / _____
                              First   Middle

Date of Admission ___ / ___ / ___   Time of Admission _____ Med. Rec. #_____
                  Mo. Day Year

Mother's Date of Birth ___ / ___ / ___ Mother's Age _____ yrs.
                       Mo. Day Year

PREGNANCY HISTORY

GTPAL / ___ / ___ / ___ / ___
        G   T   P   A   Living Children

Deceased Children _____ ☐ None

Date Last Live Birth _____ / _____
                     Mo.   Year

Terminations (spontaneous/induced)

_____ <20 Wks ☐ None

_____ ≥20 Wks ☐ None

Date Last Other Termination _____ / _____
                            Mo.   Year

CURRENT PREGNANCY

Payment for Prenatal Care and Hospitalization (Select one)
☐ 1. Private Insurance
☐ 2. Private Insurance and Self Payment
☐ 3. Medical Assistance
☐ 4. Medical Assistance and Self Payment
☐ 5. Self Payment
☐ 6. No Payment
☐ 7. Other _____
☐ 8. Medical Assistance and Private Insurance

☐ Enrolled in Prenatal Care Coordination

Month Prenatal Care Began _____ (Months 1-9)

Total No. Prenatal Visits _____ ☐ None

Last Normal Menstrual Period Began ___ / ___ / ___
                                   Mo. Day Year

Est. Date of Delivery ___ / ___ / ___
                      Mo. Day Year

Gestational Age _____ Weeks
   by: ☐ LMP ☐ Ultrasound

Blood Group _____ Rh ☐ Pos ☐ Neg

If Rh Neg, RhoGam™ 28 Wks   ☐ Yes ☐ No

Rubella Immune   ☐ Yes ☐ No

MS-AFP ☐ 1. Normal ☐ 2. High ☐ 3. Low
        ☐ 4. Not Done ☐ 5. Unknown

Weight Gained/Lost During This Pregnancy _____ (lbs.)

ANTEPARTUM MEDICAL RISK FACTORS

☐ Anemia (Hct. <30/Hgb. <10)
☐ Cardiac Disease
☐ Psychiatric Disorder
☐ Collagen Vascular Disease,
  specify _____
☐ Pre-existing Diabetes–
  Insulin Dependent
☐ Pre-existing Diabetes–
  Adult Onset
☐ Gestational Diabetes
☐ Hepatitis B
☐ Substance Use/Abuse,
  specify _____
☐ Genital Herpes
☐ Other STD's, (chlamydia,
  GC), specify _____
☐ Vaginal Infections,
  specify _____
☐ Hemoglobinopathy
☐ Hydramnios
☐ Oligohydramnios
☐ Hypertension, Chronic
☐ Hypertension, Pregnancy
  Associated
☐ Eclampsia
☐ Incompetent Cervix
☐ Lung Disease,
  Acute/Chronic
☐ Previous Infant 4000 +
  Grams

☐ Previous Preterm Infant
☐ Previous SGA Infant
☐ Renal Disease,
  specify _____
☐ Rh Sensitization
☐ Other Iso-immunization
☐ Uterine Bleeding
☐ Suspected IUGR
☐ Multiple Gestation
☐ Preterm Labor
  This Pregnancy
☐ Prolonged Preterm ROM
  (>24 hrs.)
☐ Fetal Demise
  (This Pregnancy)
☐ Fetal Compromise
  (Antenatal Testing)
☐ Diagnosed Fetal Anomaly,
  specify _____
☐ Postdatism
☐ Previous Stillbirth
☐ Urinary Tract Infections
☐ Uterine or Cervical
  Anomaly
☐ Previous C-Section
☐ None (No Risk Factors)
☐ Other,
  specify _____

ANTEPARTUM MEDICATIONS

☐ Antibiotics
☐ Anticonvulsants
☐ Antihypertensives
☐ Hormones
☐ Psychotropics
☐ Other,
  specify _____

☐ Prenatal Vitamins
☐ Prenatal Iron
☐ None

INTRAPARTUM DATA

☐ Trial of VBAC
☐ Amnionitis
☐ Blood Loss Over 500cc
☐ Febrile (>100F or 38C)
☐ Meconium, Light
☐ Meconium, Moderate,
  Heavy
☐ Premature ROM (>12 hrs.)
☐ Abruptio Placenta
☐ Placenta Previa
☐ Other Excessive Bleeding
☐ Seizures During Labor
☐ Precipitous Labor (<3 hrs.)
☐ Prolonged Labor (>20 hrs.)
☐ Prolonged ROM (>24 hrs.)
☐ Dysfunctional Labor
☐ Breech Presentation
☐ Other Malpresentation

☐ Cephalopelvic
  Disproportion/Dystocia
☐ Nuchal Cord
☐ Cord Prolapse
☐ Anesthetic Complications
☐ Fetal Distress
☐ Intrapartum Fetal Demise
☐ Uterine Atony
☐ Retained Placenta
☐ Placenta Accreta/Percreta
☐ Failure to Progress
☐ Prolonged Labor Latent
  Phase
☐ Prolonged Labor Active
  Phase
☐ Arrest Active Phase
☐ None (No Complications)
☐ Other,
  specify _____

Mother Transferred Prior To Delivery ☐ Yes ☐ No

Estimated Blood Loss _____ (cc)

INTRAPARTUM MEDICATIONS

☐ Analgesics,
  specify _____
☐ Antihypertensives
☐ Other,
  specify _____

☐ Tocolytics (I.V., this admission)
☐ Magnesium Sulfate

LABOR/OBSTETRIC DATA

Anesthesia
☐ General
☐ Epidural
  ☐ 1. Labor w/Vag Del
  ☐ 2. Labor w/C-Sec
  ☐ 3. C-Sec only
☐ Spinal
☐ Pudendal
☐ Paracervical
☐ Local
☐ Other,
  specify _____

Monitoring
☐ Electronic Fetal, Internal
☐ Electronic Fetal, External
☐ Uterine Contraction,
  Internal
☐ Uterine Contraction,
  External
☐ External Auscultation
☐ Fetal Scalp Sampling

Membranes
☐ ROM Over 24 Hrs.
☐ Clear Fluid
☐ Meconium
☐ SROM

Induction
☐ Oxytocin
☐ Artificial Rupture of
  Membranes
☐ Stimulation of Labor
☐ Prostaglandin
☐ Other,
  specify _____

Other Perinatal Procedures
☐ Amniocentesis
☐ Tocolysis
☐ Steroids
☐ Ultrasound
☐ Postpartum Sterilization
☐ Hysterectomy
☐ Other,
  specify _____

_____
_____
_____
_____
_____

☐ None

PRIMARY CARE PHYS[I]

Mother's _____

Infant's _____

ATTENDANT

Code _____

Name _____

Nurse Attendants _____

_____

Additional Attendants _____

DELIVERY

No. of Fetuses (this pregnancy) _

Birth Order (this pregnancy) ___

Presentation
☐ Vertex
☐ Breech
☐ Other, specify _____

Vaginal Delivery
☐ VBAC
☐ Spontaneous
☐ Low Forceps
☐ Mid Forceps
☐ Vacuum Extraction
☐ Asst. Breech
☐ Breech Extraction

Episiotomy/Laceration
☐ Third Degree Laceration
☐ Fourth Degree Laceration
☐ Midline
☐ Mediolateral
☐ None
☐ Other

_____
_____

BIRTH OUTCOME

☐ Live Birth   ☐ Stillbirth

☐ Out-of-Hospital Birth

Clinical Est. Gest. Age _____

Birthweight _____ lbs. ___

Crown/Heel Length _____

Apgar _____ 1 minute ___

NURSERY CARE

Admitted to (this hospital):
☐ Normal Newborn Nursery
☐ High-Risk Nursery
☐ Infant Transferred
  ☐ NICU, Name of Hospital _
    City _____
  ☐ Alternate Hospital, Name _
    City _____
  ☐ Other, specify _____
Date of Transfer _____ /
                 Mo.

MATERNAL POSTPART[UM]

☐ Maternal Death (up to 42
  days postpartum)
☐ Postpartum hemorrhage
☐ Wound infection
☐ Mastitis
☐ Endometritis
☐ Antibiotics Initiated >24 hrs
  post delivery
☐ Thromboembolic disease,
  specify _____

COMBINED MATERNAL/INFANT LOGBOOK

FIGURE 9.2 Wisconsin detailed information form.

Infant's Name _____ / _____ / _____
Last

Date of Birth ___/___/___ Time of Birth_____ Med. Rec. # _____ Sex ☐ Male
First   Mo. Day Year   Middle   Last ☐ Female

CIAN

_____
_____

_____
_____
_____
_____
_____
_____

_____of _____

Cesarean Section
☐ Primary
☐ Repeat
☐ Low Transverse
☐ Low Vertical
☐ Classical

Indication for Operative Delivery
☐ Dystocia
☐ Malpresentation
☐ Fetal Distress
☐ Malposition
☐ Patient refused trial
   of labor
☐ Other, specify_____
   _____

_ Weeks
_____ozs. or _____grams
_____in. or _____cm.
____5 minutes

_____
_____
_____
_____
___/___
Day   Year

UM COMPLICATIONS

☐ Anemia with transfusion
☐ Anemia with iron
☐ HCT <22 or Hgb <7
☐ Drop Hct >11 or Hgb >3.5
☐ Urinary tract infection
☐ None (No Complications)
☐ Other,
   specify _____

OTHER POSTPARTUM/NEONATAL INFORMATION

☐ RhoGam™ Administered   ☐ Hepatitis B Vaccine
   Postpartum (Mother)   Admininistered (Infant)
☐ Rubella Vaccine   ☐ Breast Fed
   Administered Postpartum
   (Mother)

NEONATAL DATA

☐ Assisted Ventilation <30 minutes
☐ Assisted Ventilation ≥30 minutes
☐ Oxygen Therapy >10 minutes
☐ Antibiotics
☐ Anticonvulsants
☐ Phototherapy
☐ Circumcision
☐ Transfusions
☐ Surgical Procedures, specify_____
   _____
☐ Other,specify _____
☐ None

ABNORMAL CONDITIONS OF NEWBORN

☐ Anemia (Hct <39/Hgb<13)
☐ Apnea
☐ Birth Injury/Trauma,specify _____
☐ Hemolytic Disease, specify _____
☐ Hyperbilirubinemia
☐ Hypoglycemia
☐ Hyaline Membrane Disease/RDS
☐ Hypoxic Encephalopathy
☐ Infection, specify _____
☐ Meconium Aspiration Syndrome
☐ Necrotizing Enterocolitis
☐ Seizures
☐ Trauma
☐ None (No Abnormal Conditions)
☐ Other, specify _____

CONGENITAL ABNORMALITIES OF NEWBORN

☐ Anencephalus
☐ Spina bifida/Meningocele
☐ Hydrocephalus
☐ Microcephalus
☐ Other Central Nervous System Anomalies
   specify _____
☐ Heart Malformations
☐ Other Circulatory/Respiratory Anomalies
   specify _____
☐ Rectal Atresia/Stenosis
☐ Tracheo-esophageal Fistula/Esophageal Atresia
☐ Omphalocele/Gastrochisis
☐ Other Gastrointestinal Anomalies
   specify _____
☐ Malformed Genitalia
☐ Renal Agenesis
☐ Other Urogenital Anomalies
   specify _____
☐ Cleft Lip/Palate
☐ Polydactyly/Syndactyly/Adactyly
☐ Club Foot
☐ Diaphragmatic Hernia
☐ Other Musculoskeletal/Integumental Anomaly
   specify _____
☐ Down Syndrome
☐ Other Chromosomal Anomalies
   specify _____
☐ None (No Congenital Anomalies)
☐ Other, specify _____

MATERNAL DISCHARGE

Date of Discharge ___/___/___
                  Mo. Day Year
Time of Discharge _____
Maternal Length of Stay _____Days

INFANT DISCHARGE

Infant Discharge Destination
☐ Home
☐ Transfer, specify _____
☐ Other, specify _____
Date of Discharge/Transfer ___/___/___
                           Mo. Day Year
Time of Discharge _____
Infant Length of Stay_____Days
Newborn Screen Number __ __ __ __ __ __ __

PERINATAL MORTALITY

☐ Fetal Death
☐ Neonatal Death
☐ Postneonatal Death
Date of Death ___/___/___
              Mo. Day Year
Time of Death _____
Autopsy: ☐ Yes   ☐ No
Final Diagnosis of Perinatal Death:
_____

Cause of Death	Primary	Secondary
Asphyxia	☐	☐
Blood Group Incompatibility	☐	☐
Congenital Anomaly	☐	☐
Immaturity	☐	☐
Infection	☐	☐
IUGR	☐	☐
Metabolic Disorder	☐	☐
RDS	☐	☐
Trauma	☐	☐
Other, specify_____	☐	☐

SUPPLEMENTAL INFORMATION

FIGURE 9.2 Continued.

DEPARTMENT OF HEALTH & FAMILY SERVICES
DIVISION OF HEALTH
DOH 5108 (REV. 7/96)

STATE OF WISCONSIN
Chapter 69, Wis. Stats.

HOSPITAL BIRTH WORKSHEET
(Part I Continued)

PREGNANCY HISTORY: CONFIDENTIAL INFORMATION

This information may not be viewed by the informant unless the informant is the mother or has permission from the mother to view it.

LIVE BIRTHS (exclude this child)

NOW LIVING		NOW DEAD		DATE OF LAST LIVE BIRTH Month/Year
Number ____	None ☐	Number ____	None ☐	

TERMINATIONS (spontaneous or induced)

LESS THAN 20 WKS	20 WKS OR MORE	DATE OF LAST TERMINATION Month/Year
None Number ____ ☐	None Number ____ ☐	

PRENATAL CARE		DATE LAST NORMAL	WEIGHT GAIN/LOSS
Month Care Began	No. of Visits	**MENSTRUAL** **PERIOD BEGAN:** _____ Month / Day / Year	**DURING THIS** **PREGNANCY:** _____ OR _____ Net Pounds gained / Net Pounds lost

HUSBAND'S INFORMATION:

If you are married, the husband's name and information must be given even if he is not the father of the child. **They may LATER BE REMOVED BY COURT ORDER.** The hospital must include this information, even without your permission. If you were married when the child was conceived, married between conception or birth, or married at the time of birth, then you were legally married for the purposes of completing this record. **If you are not married** you may not list the name of the father on the birth certificate. Ask for information concerning a Statement of Paternity form.

HUSBAND'S NAME - FIRST	MIDDLE	LAST	DATE OF BIRTH (Mo./Day Year)	STATE OF BIRTH (If born outside USA, name the country)

HUSBAND'S CONFIDENTIAL INFORMATION: (See Instructions below for Race, Education and Employment.)

SOCIAL SECURITY NUMBER	RACE (Specify) (White, Black, American Indian, etc.)	Is husband of Hispanic origin? Yes ☐ No ☐ If yes, specify nationality: (Mexican, Puerto Rican, Cuban, etc.)

EDUCATION*		EMPLOYMENT ONE YEAR AGO	
Elem/Second (0-12)	College (1-4 or 5+)	Occupation	Type of Firm or Agency

*Highest grade completed

RACE-Enter the race of the husband and mother on the appropriate line. Enter both races if of "mixed" race. Do not enter "Hispanic." If "Native American" enter "American Indian." If Asian or Southeast Asian, specify the national origin such as "Hmong," "Cambodian," "Chinese," "Japanese," etc.

HISPANIC ORIGIN-"Hispanic" refers to people whose origins are from Mexico, Puerto Rico, Spain, or the Spanish-speaking countries of Central or South America. If you are of hispanic origin, specify the national origin. If not of hispanic origin, check the "No" box.

EDUCATION-Enter the number of years of schooling completed. Do not count partial years (e.g., if the freshman year of college is not completed, education would be "12" under the "elementary/secondary" column). Do not include years in technical or specialty schools unless college transferable (academic) credits were received.

EMPLOYMENT ONE YEAR AGO- Enter the occupation and type of firm or agency *one year prior to this birth*. Be as specific as possible in these items (see examples below). Avoid the use of firm or agency names, instead, describe the type of business the firm or agency is involved in.

EXAMPLES:

	Occupation	Kind of Firm or Agency			Occupation	Kind of Firm or Agency
Enter:	Clerk Typist	City Health Department		Enter:	Disabled	None
Not:	Office Worker	City of Madison		Not:	Never Worked	None
				Not:	None	None
Enter:	Math Teacher	High School		Enter:	Student	High School
Not:	Teacher	Public School		Not:	None	None
Enter:	Auto Mechanic	Self-employed		Enter:	Homemaker	Own Home
Not:	Mechanic	Own		Not:	None	None
Enter:	Registered Nurse	Health Clinic		Enter:	Sales Clerk	Hardware Store
Not:	Nurse	Health Care		Not:	Clerk	Smith's Store
Enter:	Unemployed	None				
Not:	None	None				

FIGURE 9.3 Wisconsin hospital birth worksheet.

DEPARTMENT OF HEALTH & FAMILY SERVICES
DIVISION OF HEALTH
DOH 5108 (REV. 7/96)

STATE OF WISCONSIN
Chapter 69, Wis. Stats.

HOSPITAL BIRTH WORKSHEET
(Part I of II)

In order that your baby's birth certificate may be complete, accurate and acceptable for filing, the following information is required. Fill in each item carefully. Print or write legibly. Your signature is required after you have completed all items.

For Hospital use only
Mother's Medical Record Number _____
Child's Medical Record Number _____
Child's Date of Birth _____ / _____ / _____
Mo.   Day   Year
Child's Time of Birth _____
Child's sex   Male ☐   Female ☐
Data Validator _____
Data Processor _____

The items in the "Confidential Information" sections of this worksheet are available to you and to the staff of some public health and research programs who must treat it confidentially. The items are not included on a certified copy of your child's birth certificate. Social Security numbers of the parents are now required under Federal Law by the Federal Office of Child Support Enforcement. These numbers will not be retained by the State Section of Vital Statistics.

CHILD'S NAME: Enter your child's name exactly as it should appear on the birth certificate. The name entered here will be legally filed.

FIRST	MIDDLE	LAST	TITLE	DATE OF BIRTH (Month/Day/Year)

MOTHER'S INFORMATION:

MOTHER'S CURRENT NAME - FIRST	MIDDLE	LAST		

MOTHER'S BIRTH NAME - FIRST	MIDDLE	LAST	DATE OF BIRTH (Mo./Day/Year)	STATE OF BIRTH (If born outside USA, name the country)

NOTE: Mother's residence is the physical location of her home. Name the city, village or township (Minor Civil Division) in which the home is located. This is not necessarily where mail is addressed. Do not use the name of an unincorporated place.

RESIDENCE-STATE	RESIDENCE-COUNTY	RESIDENCE-INSIDE CITY, VILLAGE, TOWNSHIP	(CHECK ONE) CITY VIL TWNSH. ☐ ☐ ☐

MOTHER'S CONFIDENTIAL INFORMATION: (See instructions for Race, Education and Employment on reverse side.)

SOCIAL SECURITY NUMBER	RACE (Specify) (White, Black, American Indian, etc.)	Is the mother of Hispanic origin? ☐ Yes ☐ No If yes, specify nationality: (Mexican, Puerto Rican, Cuban, etc.)

EDUCATION*		EMPLOYMENT ONE YEAR AGO		CIGARETTE/ALCOHOL USE
Elem/Second (0-12)	College (1-4 or 5+)	Occupation	Type of Firm or Agency	Cigarette use this pregnancy? ☐ Yes ☐ No
				Avg. Number of Cigarettes Per Day _____
*Highest grade completed				Alcohol use this pregnancy? ☐ Yes ☐ No Avg. Number of Alcoholic Drinks Per Week _____

MOTHER'S MAILING ADDRESS For Birth Registration Notification STREET OR RFD CITY/VILLAGE POST OFFICE, STATE, ZIP	Social Security Number Requested by Parent? Yes ☐ No ☐	Is Mother Married? (At any time between conception and birth) Yes ☐ No ☐
☐ Check here if there is a possibility that the child may be placed for adoption. Do not enter an address if you check the box. If the address is complete, a notice will be sent to this address to inform you of the official filing of the birth certificate.	Social Security Note: If the child has been named and you request it, the State Registrar will provide to the Social Security Administration the necessary information and Social Security will send your child's social security number to the mother's mailing address.	

INFORMANT-NAME	RELATION TO CHILD

I certify that the information provided on both sides of this form is correct to the best of my knowledge and belief.

Parent/Informant Signature: _____ Date: _____

Note: Only the parent of the child can name the child or authorize the request for a social security number. If the mother is not married, she is the only parent that can do this. If the mother is married, she or her husband may sign.

(Turn over to complete second side.)

FIGURE 9.3 Continued.

the health department will most likely not accept the birth certificate for registration. A legal document cannot appear to have been altered. Computerized birth certificates allow the clerk to make changes or correct errors easily, before transmitting the final data.

PATERNITY DECLARATION

The birth certificate clerk will most likely be responsible for ensuring the completion of paternity declarations. A **paternity declaration** (Figure 9.4) is a document that legally established the paternity of a child when the mother and father are not married to each other. The father's name cannot be added to the birth certificate until the paternity declaration is signed by both parents. Establishment of paternity gives the father rights for child custody and visitation and gives the mother the right to ask the court to order the father to pay child support.

The signed paternity forms are sent by the clerk to the designated county or state office. In some states, such as North Carolina, the forms are call Paternity Affidavits and must be notarized. In California, hospitals are paid a fee for each paternity declaration signed.

BATCHING CERTIFICATES FOR MAILING

When batching birth certificates to mail to the health department, take into consideration that the envelope with the original birth certificates could be lost in the mail and never be received by the health department. In order to ensure that all births are registered, type a list (Figure 9.5) of all certificates being mailed together and enclose the list with the certificate in the envelope. A computer system may be able to print the list. Keep a copy of the list; the Health Department will return the original list with each name checked off and the date it received the certificates. If a certificate has been returned because it has been altered or an item has been omitted, this will also be noted on the master list that is returned. Once the original list has been returned, the copy may be discarded. The master lists should be kept as proof that the births were registered. The retention time frames will be determined by the health information management department director.

BIRTH CERTIFICATE LOG

In addition to processing birth certificates, the birth certificate clerk may also be responsible for maintaining the birth certificate log (Figure 9.6). The log is a list, by birth date, of all live births in the hospital. It usually gives the child's name, as determined by the parents, and the date of birth. If the last name of the mother is different from the name of the child, document the mother's name in the birth log also. If the parents are not married, the baby may be given the father's last name. But, in the MPI, the baby will probably be listed with the mother's last name and cross-referenced to the given name. The birth log is a good place to document the date the birth certificate was sent to the health department for registration. There may be no need to maintain a manual birth log with a computerized system. The log will be maintained on the system.

STATE OF CALIFORNIA - HEALTH AND HUMAN SERVICES AGENCY

CALIFORNIA DEPARTMENT OF CHILD SUPPORT SERVICES

DECLARATION OF PATERNITY

DISTRIBUTION:	ORIGINAL - DCSS
	COPY 1 & 2 - Parents
	COPY 3 - Family Support

SECTION A

Child	NAME OF CHILD - FIRST	MIDDLE	LAST
	DATE OF BIRTH	SEX	FOR STATE USE ONLY
Place of Birth	HOSPITAL NAME		CITY
	COUNTY	STATE	
Father	NAME OF FATHER - FIRST	MIDDLE	LAST
	SOCIAL SECURITY NO.	DATE OF BIRTH	PLACE OF BIRTH (STATE OR COUNTRY)
	CURRENT ADDRESS (NUMBER, STREET, CITY, ZIP)		
Mother	NAME OF MOTHER - FIRST	MIDDLE	LAST
	SOCIAL SECURITY NO.	DATE OF BIRTH	PLACE OF BIRTH (STATE OR COUNTRY)
	CURRENT ADDRESS (NUMBER, STREET, CITY, ZIP)		

SECTION B - READ OTHER SIDE BEFORE SIGNING

I declare under the penalty of perjury under the laws of the State of California that I am the biological father of the child named on this declaration and that the information provided is true and correct. I have read and understand the rights and responsibilities described on the back of this form. I understand that by signing this form I am consenting to the establishment of paternity, thereby waiving those rights. I am assuming all the rights and responsibilities of the biological father of this child. I wish to be named as the father on the child's birth certificate.

I have been orally informed of my rights and responsibilities.

I declare under the penalty of perjury under the laws of the State of California that I am the natural mother of the child named on this declaration and that the information provided is true and correct. I have read and understand the rights and responsibilities described on the back of this form. I certify that the man signing this form is the only possible father of this child. I know that by signing this form I am establishing the man signing this form as the biological father of this child with all the rights and responsibilities of a biological father under the laws of California. I consent to the establishment of paternity by signing this form.

I have been orally informed of my rights and responsibilities.

SIGNATURE OF FATHER	DATE SIGNED	SIGNATURE OF MOTHER	DATE SIGNED

SECTION C - TO BE COMPLETED BY WITNESS AT THE HOSPITAL, AGENCY OR CLINIC (PLEASE PRINT)

DECLARATION WITNESSED BY (SIGNATURE AND PRINTED NAME)	DATE

NAME OF AGENCY (HOSPITAL, CLINIC OR OTHER)

ADDRESS (ADDRESS, CITY AND ZIP CODE)

SECTION D - TO BE COMPLETED BY NOTARY PUBLIC IF NOT WITNESSED ABOVE

State of _____

County of_____

On_____before me, _____, personally

appeared_____

personally known to me (or proved to me on the basis of satisfactory evidence) to be the person(s) whose name(s) are subscribed to the within instrument and acknowledged to me that he/she/they executed the same in his/her/their signature(s) on the instrument the person(s), or the entity on behalf of which the person(s) acted, executed the instrument.

WITNESS by hand and official seal.

CS 909 (1/00)

FIGURE 9.4 Paternity declaration.

```
┌─────────────────────────────────────────────┐
│                                             │
│   Mercy Medical Center                      │
│                                             │
│   5/11/2XXX                                 │
│                                             │
│      1.   Jacobs, Jane Marie      5/6/2XXX  │
│      2.   Miller, Susan Kaye      5/7/2XXX  │
│      3.   Jones, David Allen      5/9/2XXX  │
│      4.   O'Brien, Patrick Kelly  5/9/2XXX  │
│                                             │
│                                             │
└─────────────────────────────────────────────┘
```

FIGURE 9.5 List of birth certificates being submitted to the Health Department.

COMPLIMENTARY BIRTH CERTIFICATES

Many hospitals give their new mothers complimentary birth certificates. These are usually preprinted on card stock with the hospital's logo and may be signed by the hospital administrator or the Obstetrics nursing supervisor. The complimentary certificate is intended to be memento for the family. It is often used as proof of the birth when applying for Medicaid benefits for the baby.

The birth certificate clerk may be required to fill out the certificate with information such as the baby's name, date and time of birth, birth weight and length, and the names of the parents.

NEWBORN TEST RESULTS

Laboratory tests that can be performed on newborns will indicate a potential for developmental problems and diseases. If the state has a mandatory testing law, it is usually the HIM department's responsibility to ensure that the results of the laboratory test(s) are filed in the newborn's medical record. One way to track receipt of the test results is to mark the receipt date in the birth log next to the child's name (Figure 9.6). Periodically, the birth log should be checked for those newborns who have not had test results received. The department will have a procedure developed for notifying the pediatrician or the state organization conducting the test that the results have

No.	Name	DOB	Date to Health Dept.	Newborn Test Results Date
23.	JACOBS, Jane Marie	5/6/2XXX	5/11	5/20
24.	MILLER, Susan Kaye	5/7/2XXX	5/11	5/22
25.	JONES, David Allen Mother—Karen Smith	5/9/2XXX	5/11	5/25
26.	O'BRIEN, Patrick Kelly	5/9/2XXX	5/11	5/25

FIGURE 9.6 Birth log.

not been received. If the birth log is computerized, it may be necessary to use some other means of tracking receipt of newborn test results.

$\mathcal{T}$RANSCRIPTION CLERK

The function of the transcription clerk is to provide the clerical support necessary to keep dictated reports moving and transcriptionists typing. For purposes of describing this function, we will assume that the health information management department uses a digital dictation system. In a department using a tank or digital system, the duties of the transcription clerk will vary somewhat.

When a physician dictates into a digital **dictation system,** the dictation is stored on a computer hard drive. The system has a management component (Figure 9.7) that assigns each dictation a job number and records the date and time of dictation, the report type, and the dictating physician's ID number. The system also shows which transcriptionist is working on the report.

Verification

One of the most important functions of a transcription clerk is to verify that the patient demographic information on transcribed reports is accurate. **Transcription systems** have an error queue where a report will go when data fields on the report, such as name and medical record number, don't match the data fields in the ADT system. The clerk's job is to check each report in the queue, determine which field(s) is in error, make the correction(s), and then print the report. Often such errors occur when there are home-based transcriptionists who may not always have access to the ADT system and can't do their own verification.

Job No.	Author	Trans.	Auth Date	Trans Date	Status	Subject	WrkType	Dept	Job Length
61	595		05-19/14:19		Ci	320800	9		00:00:07
16	595		05-19/14:24		C	32080042	9		00:00:17
62	595		05-19/14:24		Ci	32080042	9		00:00:17
17	595		05-19/14:25		C	320800	9		00:00:11
18	595		05-20/09:45		C	32080024	9		00:00:00
19	595		05-20/09:46		C	32080024	9		00:00:06
20	595		05-20/09:47		C	32080024	9		00:00:03
21	595		05-20/09:47		C	32080014	9		00:00:00
22	595		05-20/10:02		C	32080014	9		00:00:08
23	595		05-20/10:02		C	32080024	9		00:00:03
24	595		05-20/10:03		C	32080024	9		00:00:00
25	595		05-20/10:08		C	32080024	9		00:00:00
26	595		05-20/10:09		C	320800	9		00:00:04
27	595		05-20/10:13		C	320800	9		00:00:00
28	595		05-20/15:10		C	32080059	9		00:00:00
29	595		05-20/15:13		C	32080059	9		00:00:00
30	595		05-20/16:07		C		9		00:00:00
31	595		05-20/16:09		C	9	9		00:00:04
32	595		05-20/16:12		C	320800	9		00:00:04
33	595		05-20/16:14		C	41608	9		00:00:07
34	595		05-20/16:24		C	41608	9		00:00:00
35	595		05-20/16:24		C	4160824	9		00:00:04
36	595		05-20/16:32		C	32080024	9		00:00:10
37	595		05-20/17:00		C	4160824	9		00:00:35
38	595		05-21/12:33		C	9712140	9		00:00:26

VoicePower 2000 User Interface - [Work Status Window]
File Edit Marked Jobs View Window Help
VoicePower 2000   Status Codes   Custom Setting

Jobs	Length	Tot Jobs	Tot Len	Page	Update Progress	Marked Jobs	Auth Time	Trans Time
68	00:13:12	68	00:13:12	2 of 3	100%	0	01:23:24	00:00:00

View 1	Show Names	Record Filter	Update Now!	Page Up	Page Down

For Help, press F1   NUM

FIGURE 9.7 A digital dictation system management screen (courtesy Digital Voice, Inc.).

Print and Deliver Reports

Transcription systems allow the transcriptionist to specify the number of copies of each report to be printed. Each copy prints separately, so the clerk does not have to sort pages. The clerk then staples each copy and delivers one to the nursing unit. Some hospitals have the capability of printing directly to nursing units and outpatient clinics, eliminating the need for report delivery.

Physician copies are often faxed directly to the physician's office. The transcription system has a fax server with a database of the physician fax numbers and the time of day each wants his or her reports faxed. This is usually at night, so that the fax machine is not tied up during the day when it is needed for other uses.

Monitor Transcription and Dictation Systems

Digital dictation and transcription systems require consistent monitoring. The clerk must insure that all reports have printed and that any reports that have been put on hold for any reason are not forgotten and never released to print. The clerk may put reports on hold so the supervisor can conduct quality checks, and then must release them for printing.

The transcription clerk assigns work to home-based transcriptionists using the digital dictation management system. He or she monitors the dictation system to insure that reports that have been transcribed are being archived, so the system doesn't fill up. A digital system will not record over dictation already on the system, but it can fill up and not be able to record additional dictation.

The clerk adds new physician information, including the dictation ID number into the dictation system so that the physician will be able to access the system and dictate.

The interface between the dictation system and the transcription system is monitored by the transcription clerk, to insure that the transcriptionists will receive the data entered by physicians when dictating.

The fax server is monitored to make sure all faxed reports went through to the receiving physician's office. If a report did not go through, perhaps because the physician's fax machine was malfunctioning or out of paper, the clerk resends the fax.

The dial-in computers connecting the home-based transcriptionists to the transcription system are monitored by the clerk to ensure they are functioning.

Some hospitals have an interface between the transcription system and a hospital-wide mainframe computer. The interface must be monitored by the clerk to insure all documents make it to the mainframe.

Contract Services

Many hospitals utilize contract transcription services to help maintain acceptable transcription turnaround times and to insure that the dictation system does not fill up. If the service has the equipment to dial into the dictation system, the transcription clerk assigns the reports to the service's transcriptionists, using the management functions.

The clerk monitors the work assigned to the service, making sure all reports get transcribed, and then imports the transcribed reports into the hospital's transcription system, performs verification, and prints the reports.

If the service cannot dial in, the clerk may have to rerecord the dictation onto the service's dictation system, over phone lines, or, in a worst-case scenario, rerecord

CONTRACT SERVICE LOG					
Job #	Report	Patient	Physician	MR #	Date
1356	OP	Landry, Anna	Smith	06-75-02	5/14
1357	DS	Morgan, Marlene	Miller	05-37-19	5/10-5/15
1359	H&P	Hernandez, Alma	Beaudette	06-75-50	5/16
1360	Cons	Hernandez, Alma	Smith	06-75-50	5/16
1361	Proc	Hernandez, Alma	Beaudette	06-75-50	5/16

FIGURE 9.8 Contract transcription service log.

the dictation onto cassettes. Rerecording onto cassettes is a real-time function (i.e., it takes eight hours to rerecord eight hours of dictation).

When cassettes are sent to a contract service, it is necessary to keep a **transcription log** of the reports sent out (Figure 9.8). The log will contain the dictation system job number, report type, correct spelling of the patient's name, the patient's medical record number, the physician's name, and the dates of treatment. The log is useful, when the transcribed reports are returned, in ensuring that all reports have been received.

Customer Service

While performing all of his or her other duties, the transcription clerk is responsible for answering the phone and helping customers. Customer requests include faxing reports to physician offices, helping physicians who are having problems dictating, and locating copies of reports for nursing units.

TRANSCRIPTION LOG						
Date Dictated	Physician Name	Patient Name	Report Type	Date Trans.	Line Count	TI
6/1	Jones, T.	Andrews, David	DS	6/2	97	KM
	Mallon	Smith, James	OP	6/1	76	GB
6/2	Keefer	Plitt, Amanda	H&P	6/2	77	KM
	Jackson	Plitt, Amanda	Cons	6/2	81	KM

FIGURE 9.9 Transcription log.

Noncomputerized Systems

In hospitals with no or partial computerization, the transcription clerk may be responsible for maintaining a manual report log (Figure 9.9), sorting and stapling reports and copies, delivering reports to nursing units, and mailing copies to physician offices periodically.

Concurrent Monitoring of Dictation

Another function that may be conducted by the transcription clerk is concurrent monitoring of H&P and operative report dictation. The JCAHO requires that H&Ps and operative reports be dictated within 24 hours of admission and immediately after surgery, respectively. This monitoring may be done by taking the daily admission list and the surgery schedule and checking them against the transcription log.

CASE MANAGEMENT CLERK

The case management clerk assists the case managers by setting up the daily workload of inpatient records to be reviewed. He or she sorts the faxed requests for reviews from insurance companies and picks other patients for review based on established protocols. There may be protocols requiring review for specific diagnoses, length of stay, focus areas in the hospital, and particular DRGs.

During the day, the clerk is responsible for monitoring requests received by fax; these can number 50 to 60 per day or more at a busy hospital. The case management clerk is also responsible for opening mail and responding to requests for retrospective reviews and denials of payment by insurance companies. The first step for each is to request the medical record from the health information management department. If the retrospective review request is made more than a few months after discharge, the clerk may be responsible for sending the requestor copies of the medical record rather than having a case manager take time away from inpatient reviews.

With denial responses, the case management clerk will obtain the record and determine the patient's length of stay, physician name, treating service (e.g., Med/Surg), and the total charges for the episode of care. This information and the record are then given to the case manager, who decides whether the denial will be appealed. If so, the case management clerk will type the appeal letter and copy the pertinent portions of the record. The clerk logs all denials and tracks the appeals process for each.

CANCER REGISTRY CLERK

As stated in Chapter 2, a cancer registry is a database of patients diagnosed with cancer. Data are compiled on each patient from the time the original diagnosis is made through any treatment or related therapy for the cancer. Information collected includes patient demographic data, date of initial diagnosis, primary site of tumor, site or sites of additional tumors, and dates and types of treatment. The cancer registry clerk may assist in case finding and collecting data and will be responsible for achieving the required 90 percent follow-up of patients annually. Case finding involves reviewing lists of new patients for suspected cancer symptoms or diagnoses, reviewing diagnosis codes assigned, reviewing pathology reports, or reviewing physician office

MEDICAL CENTER

10/19/

DR

The Cancer Registry is doing our yearly follow-up on this patient. We would appreciate it if you would fill out the information below.

PATIENT:
DATE OF BIRTH: 10/08/1950

DATE OF DIAGNOSIS: /04/11
SITE: LYMPH NODE - NOS
ML LARGE CELL DI

DATE OF YOUR LAST PATIENT CONTACT:

      ____/____/____

STATUS AT LAST CONTACT:
_____ Alive no evidence of this cancer
_____ Alive with evidence of this cancer
_____ Dead
       •Date of death ____/____/____
       •Cause _____

QUALITY OF SURVIVAL:
_____ Normal activity
_____ Symptomatic and ambulatory
_____ Ambulatory more than 50%, occasionally
       needs assistance
_____ Ambulatory less than 50%, nursing care
       needed
_____ Bedridden, may require hospitalization
_____ Unknown / unspecified

If you are not currently following the patient, please indicate a physician whom we may contact for follow-up information:

_____

_____

DATE OF LAST FOLLOW-UP: /09/09

PATIENT'S CURRENT ADDRESS:

Please indicate a change in patient's address here:

_____

_____

FIRST RECURRENCE:

Date ___/___/___

Site(s) _____

SUBSEQUENT TREATMENT / DATES:
Surgery _____ ___/___/___

Radiation _____ ___/___/___

Chemotherapy _____ ___/___/___

Hormonal _____ ___/___/___

Other _____ ___/___/___

METASTASIS:
____ Yes   Site(s) _____
____ No

FIGURE 9.10 Cancer registry follow-up letter.

billing data. To conduct follow-up, the clerk will contact (Figure 9.10) physicians' offices, other healthcare facilities, and the patient to document the patient's condition since the last follow-up contact. Follow-up is continued annually through life.

OUTPATIENT CLINIC CLERK

Large medical centers often operate their own outpatient clinics, where patients see their physicians. When a clinic is operated under the hospital's license, the health information management department has responsibility for maintaining and providing records for the clinic. Outpatient clinic records may be filed in separate file folders or they may be found in the same folder as the inpatient record. If the outpatient record is filed separately, it may be the clerk's responsibility to obtain the inpatient record when it is requested by the caregiver.

The outpatient clinic clerk is responsible for pulling the records of scheduled patients from the files. This is usually done several days before the scheduled appointment, so that the clinic nursing staff has time to check the record and make sure that the results of all tests and any dictations from the previous visit are filed in the record. This process is called chart prep. In some hospitals, the clinic clerk is responsible for chart prep.

Other duties of the clerk include loose report filing, creation and repair of file folders, refiling records, and searching for missing records. Outpatient clinic records usually have a set of dividers to separate such forms as progress notes, lab reports, orders, and the like. Forms are usually filed in reverse chronological order behind the appropriate divider.

OPTICAL IMAGING CLERK

Hospitals that use optical imaging to store their medical records have found a solution to many of the greatest challenges in maintaining paper records. An imaged record can be viewed by multiple users at the same time in different locations. Once a record has been scanned and indexed properly, the possibility of misfiles and lost records is virtually eliminated.

The optical imaging clerk's job is the first step in making a record available on an imaging system. The paper record is received in the health information management department from the patient care areas, as usual. Instead of assembling the record, however, it is prepped for scanning. This means that all staples are removed, any torn or crumpled pages are repaired, and (depending on the imaging system) pages are placed in chronological order.

Once prepped, the documents are batched and scanning begins. The scanner looks like a copy machine. High-speed scanners have a sheet feeder that automatically pulls each page into the scanner. Flatbed scanners require that each page be individually placed. Before starting the scanner, the clerk enters the batch number into the computer attached to the scanner.

Once the batch has been scanned, the clerk begins indexing. Each document that has been successfully scanned is shown, one by one, on the computer screen. To one side are fields that must be filled in to identify the document type, patient name, case number, and medical record number. If the form is barcoded (see Figure 5.12), the document type fills in automatically. If not, the clerk can select the type from a list on the computer. The clerk may also be able to indicate, on the computer, when the patient information is the same for successive documents. This eliminates the clerk's having to enter the demographics for every page.

Once indexing is complete, the clerk releases the batch to a quality control queue. Quality control (QC) may be performed on 100 percent of the images. The clerk compares each paper page with the imaged page to insure that it is legible and that it has been indexed correctly. Sometimes a page will be crumpled during the scanning process or a document is indexed with the wrong document type. The QC clerk returns the paper pages to be rescanned or indexed. If these errors are not corrected, either the page will be unreadable or a user will not be able to find the document he or she is looking for without paging through the entire record. A document indexed to the wrong patient is the same as filing a paper document in the wrong file folder. Once released from QC, the record may be viewed by users. The paper record is boxed and eventually destroyed.

Prepping, scanning, indexing, and quality control may be separate functions performed by different optical imaging clerks, or each clerk may be responsible for all.

SUMMARY

The medical records/HIM clerk has an important role in processing birth certificates and monitoring the work produced by transcriptionists. Alternative roles in cancer registry, case management, outpatient clinics, and optical imaging offer diversity in choosing a career path.

LEARNING ACTIVITIES

1. True or False:
   __ The format of a birth certificate is standard across the country.
   __ A birth certificate may be corrected as long as the correction cannot be seen.
   __ When a birth certificate is amended, the original birth certificate is changed to show the new information.
   __ It is important to keep a list of the birth certificates sent to the health department until verification of receipt has been received.
   __ The paternity declaration must be signed by only the father of the baby.
   __ The paternity declaration legally establishes paternity of the baby.
   __ The complimentary birth certificate can be used as proof of the birth.
   __ A manual birth log must be maintained with a computerized birth certificate system.
   __ The cancer registry clerk codes all tumors.

2. Define transcription verification and why it is so important.

3. What are the different methods a hospital may use in making dictation available to a contract service?

4. What is the percentage of follow-up required of a cancer registry? How does the clerk conduct follow-up?

5. What is the case management clerk's role in responding to denials of payment?

6. Define chart prep as it pertains to an outpatient clinic record.

7. Describe the four functions performed by an optical imaging clerk.

Bibliography

California Healthcare Association. *Consent Manual,* Current Edition. California Healthcare Association, Sacramento, California.

Huffman, EK. *Health Information Management,* 10th Edition. Physicians Record Company, Berwyn, Illinois.

Joint Commission on Accreditation of Healthcare Organizations. *Accreditation Manual for Hospitals,* Current Edition. Joint Commission on Accreditation of Healthcare Organizations, Chicago, Illinois.

Joint Commission on Accreditation of Healthcare Organizations. *Hospital Accreditation Program Scoring Guidelines, Medical Staff Standards,* Current Edition. Joint Commission on Accreditation of Healthcare Organizations, Chicago, Illinois.

Index

(continued)